MEASUREMENT IN ANAESTHESIA

BOERHAAVE SERIES
FOR POSTGRADUATE
MEDICAL EDUCATION
Nr. 9

PROCEEDINGS OF THE BOERHAAVE COURSES
ORGANIZED BY
THE FACULTY OF MEDICINE, UNIVERSITY OF LEIDEN
THE NETHERLANDS

MEASUREMENT
IN
ANAESTHESIA

EDITED BY

S.A. FELDMAN M.D., J.M. LEIGH M.D. AND JOH. SPIERDIJK M.D.

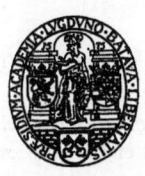

LEIDEN UNIVERSITY PRESS
1974

Library of Congress Catalog Card Number 74-83805

ISBN-13:978-94-010-2322-1   e-ISBN-13:978-94-010-2320-7
DOI: 10.1007/978-94-010-2320-7

Jacket design: E. Wijnans

© 1974 Leiden University Press, Leiden, The Netherlands
Softcover reprint of the hardcover 1st edition 1974

PREFACE

The 1973 Boerhaave Course in Leiden on Measurement in Anaesthesia was composed of the lectures included in this book, supplemented by the series of 'lecture demonstrations' organised by Dr. P. Cliffe and given by the members of the Departments of Clinical Measurement and the Magill Department of Anaesthetics, Westminster Hospital, London.

The aim of the 1973 Boerhaave Course on Measurement in Anaesthesia was designed to arouse interest in this subject where it has not already occurred.

The subjects discussed in the lectures and presented in this book were those that were considered topical and appropriate. The lectures were meant to give an idea of some basic and advanced possibilities of measurement. It was not intended to be an exhaustive review of all the measurements relevant to anaesthetic practice and research. In this time of monitoring one has to keep in mind that good measurement is the basis of good monitoring.

A certain amount of repetition is unavoidable as each lecture was intended to be complete in itsel. However, editing has reduced this to a minimum.

Department of Anaesthesiology   Johan Spierdijk
University Hospital, Leiden

Department of Anaesthetics   Stanley Feldman
Westminster Hospital, London   Julian Leigh

CONTENTS

PART TWO
MEASUREMENT OF RESPIRATORY AND ANAESTHETIC GASES

PART THREE
MEASUREMENT OF THE CIRCULATION

CONTENTS

PART FOUR
COMPUTERS

CONTRIBUTORS

J. E. W. BENEKEN, Institute of Medical Physics TNO, Utrecht, The Netherlands.

J. P. BLACKBURN, Department of Clinical Measurement, Westminster Hospital, London, U.K.

A. G. L. BURM, Department of Anaesthesiology, University Hospital, Leiden, The Netherlands.

M. S. CHRISTENSEN, Department of Anaesthesiology, Bispebjerg Hospital, Copenhagen, Denmark.

P. CLIFFE, Department of Clinical Measurement, Westminster Hospital, London, U.K.

C. CONWAY, Magill Department of Anaesthesiology, Westminster Medical School, University of London, U.K.

J. C. DORLAS, Department of Anaesthesiology, University Hospital, Groningen, The Netherlands.

H. J. EIKENBROEK, Department of Clinical Psychology, University of Leiden, The Netherlands.

S. A. FELDMAN, Magill Department of Anaesthesiology, Westminster Medical School, University of London, U.K.

P. J. JANSSEN, Department of Anaesthesiology, University Hospital, Leiden, The Netherlands.

A. LACK, Department of Clinical Measurement, Westminster Hospital, London, U.K.

J. M. LEIGH, Magill Department of Anaesthesiology, Westminster Medical School, University of London, U.K.

H. MATTIE, Departments of Pharmacology and Internal Medicine, University Hospital, Leiden, The Netherlands.

G. ROLLY, Department of Anaesthesiology, University Hospital, Gent, Belgium.

JOH. SPIERDIJK, Department of Anaesthesiology, University Hospital, Leiden, The Netherlands.

K. STEINBEREITHNER, Institut für Anaesthesiologie, Universität von Wien, Osterreich.

M. K. SYKES, Department of Anaesthetics, Royal Postgraduate Medical School, University of London, U.K.

K. H. WESSELING, Institute of Medical Physics TNO, Utrecht, The Netherlands.

PART ONE

INTRODUCTION

THE DIFFERENCE BETWEEN MEASUREMENT AND MONITORING
WHAT IS WORTH MEASURING?

JOH. SPIERDIJK AND A. NANDORFF

Today anaesthesiology is in the process of changing from a simple profession concerned with the administration of anaesthetics to a complex field with many sub-specialties. The patient we treat is committed to our care and we shall help and support him in every way we can. During treatment, the patient can depend upon our experience, our insight, our clinical know-how and our well-educated hand. He is thankful for this care and attention. But there is more – later the patient will want to express his thanks for this care and he must be able to do so! That is why he must receive expert treatment. The competence of the anaesthetist is formed by his general medical knowledge and his specific knowledge of anaesthesiology. This knowledge rests to a large extent on basic subjects such as pharmacology, physiology, mathematics, statistics and measurement.

The patient can also profit from an anaesthetists' specialized knowledge in a specific field such as cardio-anaesthesiology, neuro-anaesthesiology, intensive care and the pain clinic. Although it is possible at present for an anaesthetist to be active in all branches of this field, I believe that in the future anaesthesiology must be divided into sub-specialties – certainly in the teaching centres. There students and future specialists can acquire the specific knowledge inherent in these sub-specialties while the patient can profit from the advanced medical care.

Supervision of the patient with so-called monitoring equipment occurs in most modern hospitals. Here we understand monitoring to mean continuous visualization of the measurement of a specific phenomenon. This measurement is visualized on a scale, screen or writer. It can also be stored on tape or in a computer for later re-call. Limits can be set beforehand; if the limit is exceeded, for instance, alarm is given.

The basis of good monitoring is good measurement. Measurement is the assignment of numbers to represent properties according to rules. We

3

anaesthetists are interested in measurement – not only to obtain good monitoring but also to increase our knowledge and insight into anaesthesiology.
Not only our senses but also our intellect must provide insight into the
essence of anaesthesiology, and must teach us the influence of anaesthetics
on vital functions, metabolic processes, electrolyte shifts and enzyme reactions. For this purpose, measurement is necessary in the laboratory, but
also before, during and after anaesthesia. To be sure we understand one
another correctly, I do not mean that we must ignore our feelings while
treating a patient.

After successful operation, our patient must be able to deliver the same
(or better) physical and cerebral performance as beforehand. His psychological balance may not be disturbed. These factors are the measure of success
for anaesthesiology, independent of all processes involved, independent too
of what we do or do not measure. We of course assume hereby that recovery
occurs within a very short time after surgery (1).

Many of the phenomena which are important during anaesthesia are
easily measured. The value of the measurement of an arbitrary phenomenon
depends on the situation. In research measurement will probably be more
extensive than in clinical practice. During clinical practice, the situation
determines what is to be measured. In all cases, it is necessary to be aware
of the reliability of the measurement. Knowledge of the different methods
of measurement is also essential; furthermore use of a certain method should
not be avoided just because it is not routine procedure in that particular
department. During cardiosurgery, for instance, electrolyte shifts are followed with precision; this should also be the case during many of the other
long, major operations. The following phenomena are routinely monitored
during neurosurgery:

   blood pressure
   pulse rate
   ECG and finger plethysmogram
   central venous pressure
   blood loss
   urine excreted
   alveolar pCO_2
   respiratory, tidal and minute volumes.
When the danger of an air embolism necessitates close observation, an
oesphageal stethoscope and a right atrial catheter are also used.

In a specific study of the induced hypotensive anaesthesia technique, we
measure and record intra-arterial blood pressure. In addition we take

arterial samples regularly for estimation of pCO_2, bicarbonate, O_2 saturation, PO_2, base excess, and lactate and pyruvate levels.

During surgery for cerebral aneurysms or vascular meningiomas, deliberate hypotension is often indicated. A risk of this technique is hypoxia of the cerebral tissue. There is no simple answer to the question: what is a safe arterial PO_2 (2). A large number of interacting factors determines the cellular PO_2 (acid-base balance, Hb, CBF).

Changes in serum lactate concentration and the lactate/pyruvate ratio may be early signs of oxygen deficiency. The metabolic demands of the brain are high (3). The currency of energy is ATP. ATP is formed from ADP and inorganic phosphate. The fuel which supplies the energy for ATP synthesis is glucose. Most of the glucose is first converted to pyruvic acid (by the glycolytic pathway); ATP is then formed via a series of oxidative reactions in the Krebs cycle. Each mole of glucose produces 38 moles of ATP.

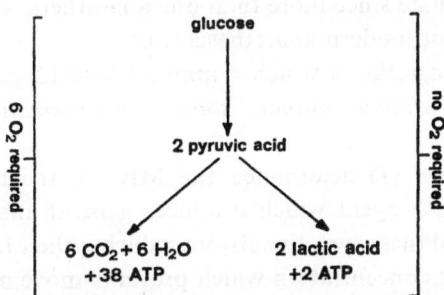

Fig. 1. From: Neurologic considerations. Clinical Anaesthesia Series, p.8, M.H. Harmel (ed.), Blackwell Scientific Publications, Oxford 1967.

The absence of oxygen causes reversion to the more primitive anaerobic (glycolytic) pathway whereby glucose is converted to lactic acid. If there is glycolysis, then only 2 moles of ATP are formed from each mole of glucose. Anaerobic synthesis of ATP is therefore not sufficient to maintain a normal cerebral function. Tissue hypoxia increases the rate of glycolysis and thus lactate production. Elevated lactate levels alone do not justify the conclusion that there is tissue hypoxia (4). An increase in lactate also occurs during alkalosis due to hypocarbia; in this case, however, the pyruvate levels are also elevated. The L/P ratio is a more reliable indicator of anaerobic metabolism (5).

In alkalosis the L/P ratio is unchanged; in hypoxia, it increases. Therefore blood gas analyses should be carried out together with the lactate/pyruvate measurements. The relationship between the direction of change (increase or decrease) in lactate concentration and the L/P ratio will indicate the correct interpretation. Hypoxia is probably the only condition with the combination of increased lactate plus increased L/P ratio (4).

Normal values: lactate in arterial blood: 0.5 — 1.5 mmole/l
                        pyruvate in arterial blood: 0.05 — 0.15 mmole/l
Physiological L/P ratio = 10.

DEPTH OF ANAESTHESIA

An increasing number of authors have indicated their interest in finding a method of measurement suitable for comparing the anaesthesiological action of various anaesthetic agents by means of comparable concentrations. The depth of anaesthesia was first defined by Guedel, who introduced the classical scheme for the clinical signs of nervous depression. Today, however, his approach is inadequate since more than one anaesthetic agent is required to meet the demands of modern anaesthesia (6).

A definition of anaesthesia which is applicable to all general anaesthetics is: *unconsciousness without unwanted somatic or automatic reactions to surgical stimuli.*

Furthermore Snow (7) determined the MIC or the minimum inspired concentration of each agent which produces general anaesthesia. In 1965 Eger et al. combined these two, thereby introducing the MAC: the minimum alveolar anaesthetic concentration which prevents movement in response to a standard stimulus (= surgical incision) (8). This concept, which was soon assimilated in practice, has several important advantages:

1. a new objectivity is introduced in the thinking of the anaesthetist;
2. the anaesthetic level can be expressed intelligibly;
3. calculation of a therapeutic index for anaesthetic agents is now possible. Some MAC values are:

	vol %
nitrous oxide	101.0
cyclopropane	9.2
diethyl ether	1.92
halothane	0.765
methoxyflurane	0.16

If we substitute arterial for alveolar in MAC, then it is applicable for the non-volatile anaesthetic agents.

Lately several other abbreviations have been introduced. We should remember that we are considering an E.D.$_{50}$.

MIC   =   Minimum inspired concentration
MAC   =   Minimum alveolar concentration
MArC   =   Minimum arterial concentration
CUNC   =   Concentration which causes unconsciousness
CME   =   Concentration of maximum efficacy
MAC$_{awake}$ =   Concentration at which a patient first regains conscious-
                   ness.

The CME prevents a reaction to the severest surgical stimuli, such as mesenteric traction or forceful rectal dilatation. Originally Marken, Faulconer and Bickford assumed that all general anaesthetics yield a basically similar dose-dependent sequence of six different electroencephalographic patterns. Later, it appeared that some anaesthetics do not produce every electroencephalographic pattern in the basic sequence and that a particular pattern did not necessarily signify the same clinical state for different drugs.

In modern practice, estimation of the depth of anaesthesia has become less important. General anaesthetics are administered in relatively low concentrations since the use of muscle relaxants eliminates somatic reactions to surgery. It is of great interest, however, to investigate the different neurophysiological effects of the different agents.

It was demonstrated that the structure of an anaesthetic is closely related to its sensory evoked responses and EEG-effects (9). Average Sensory Evoked Responses provide a new neurophysiological method for comparing the effects of different anaesthetics in man and animals. Both the EEG and SER patterns are determined by the chemical structure of an anaesthetic drugs. The different patterns should express different regional actions in the brain (reticular formation, non-specific thalamus, cerebral cortex). The clinical states which mark general anaesthesia probably do not require every action which an anaesthetic exerts on the brain.

The measurement of drug concentrations and the use of standard methods for assessing neurophysiological changes are recommended for future investigation of new agents. To organize the results of new studies, a classification of volatile agents is given (table 1) V.

TEMPERATURE

The measurement of temperature is exceedingly important in surgical patients (11). The environment of the modern operating room is cool (19–21°C)

CHEMICAL GROUP

INORGANIC AGENTS	HYDROCARBONS	FOUR-CARBON ETHERS	THREE-CARBON ETHERS	HALOGENATED HYDROCARBONS	INCREASING CNS IRRITABILITY
XENON XE	CYCLOPROPANE $CH_2CH_2CH_2$	DIETHYL ETHER $CH_3CH_2OCH_2CH_3$	METHOXY-FLURANE $CH_3OCF_2CHCl_2$	TRICHLOROETHYLENE $CHCl:CCl_2$	→
NITROUS OXIDE N_2O		FLUROXENE $CF_3CH_2OCH:CH_2$	FORANE $CHF_2OCHClCF_3$	HALOTHANE CHLOROFORM $CHClBrCF_3$ $CHCl_3$	
			ENFLURANE CHF_2OCF_2CHFCl		

Tabel 1. Classification of inhalational agents. D.L. After Clark and B. S. Rosner (6).

with low relative humidity and is regulated for the comfort of the surgical team (12 13) but not for the patient.

PERCENTAGE COMFORTABLE

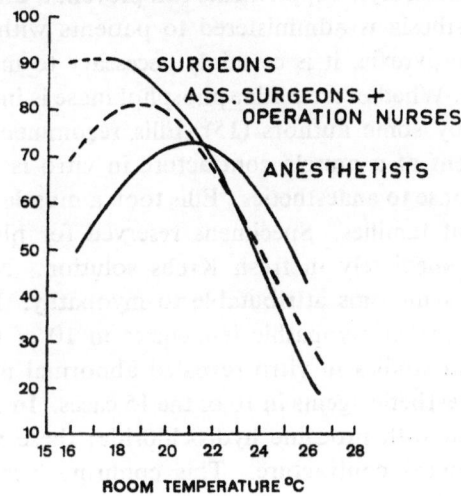

Fig. 2.

The unconscious patient cannot reveal his feelings. Usually when the skin temperature falls below 33 °C, heat production is stimulated and oxygen consumption increases. There is a critical core temperature between 35.5 and 37.2 °C. Shivering during anaesthesia is rare unless there is a rapid, sharp drop in temperature during light anaesthesia; and the fact that loss of body heat occurs during anaesthesia suggests that compensatory mechanisms are impaired.

After surgery, restlessness, shivering and an increase in oxygen consumption may be noted. This rise in oxygen consumption may coincide with hypoxia due to the after-effects of anaesthesia and shivering must therefore be avoided.

The measurement of a high temperature during and after anaesthesia is also highly significant. In additon to fever due to various causes, the patient may suffer from either hyperthermia due to shock and dehydration (13) or the so-called malignant hyperpyrexia (14).

Hyperthermia due to shock and dehydration is characterized by a fluid deficiency or a storage of extra-cellular fluids. In both cases, the body is not able to cool off because of the decreased circulation in the skin and diminished perspiration. Loss of heat is therefore insufficient.

Measurement of temperature and volume of urine excreted in conjunction with fluid and electrolyte supplements can prevent a dramatic hyperthermia.

Before anaesthesia is administered to patients with a family history of malignant hyperpyrexia, it is certainly necessary to measure the creatinine phosphokinase. Whether creatinine phosphokinase is indeed a good measure is questioned by some authors (15). Ellis recommends a muscle biopsy. The development of a muscle contracture in vitro is considered a specific abnormal response to anaesthetics. Ellis took a muscle biopsy in 18 patients from 8 different families. Specimens reserved for pharmacological study were placed immediately in fresh Krebs solution. None of the patients complained of symptoms attributable to myopathy. Nevertheless histological studies revealed myopathic tendencies in 10 of the first 15 patients; pharmacological studies in vitro revealed abnormal muscle activity in the presence of anaesthetic agents in 10 of the 15 cases. In 3 patients, the muscle was first treated with procaine hydrochloride; these preparations did not develop the typical contracture. This confirms, according to Ellis, the reasoning behind procaine treatment.

COMPUTERS

It is today a tactical assumption that many facets of clinical medicine require computer assistance to manipulate the quantitative clinical measurements. The strategic question is whether the clinical measurements involved warrent – in the long run – the outlay in money and effort. Sayers (16) is not optimistic about the use of computers in clinical medicine except under special circumstances. According to him, the hypothetical advantages of a computer system for patient supervision are valid in, for example, cardiac intensive care or post-thoracic surgery. I believe that in the near future we shall depend on the computer not only for clinical measurement but also to predict the values we need. I hope to hear more about this type of development from our last group of speakers.

In conclusion I would like to consider briefly the complications and our responsibility. If, for example we wish to compare the CO_2 content of the end-expiratory with the PCO_2 in arterial blood, we should realize that puncture of the radial artery can lead to thrombosis and aneurysms (18, 19, 20). Downs et al. (17) state that catheters with the largest external diameter relative to the size of the vessel are associated with the highest rate of vascular occlusion and thrombosis formation. Bedford and Wollman (18) report that 40% of the radial artery punctures result in thrombosis.

In all cases, however, there was recanalization. These articles indicate that before a catheter is inserted in the radial artery, we should be sure that the ulnar artery can handle the blood supply (20). This example can be followed by various others.

We must be aware of the complications threatening the patients as a result of our methods of measurement. That our electronic measuring apparatures can be dangerous is the subject of the next paper. I believe that we meet our responsibility if we know why we measure, and if we know what complications can occur. We are as anaesthetists used to accepting responsibility – but it is good for us to realize that we are also responsible for the complications which can result from unnecessary or incorrectly executed measurement.

Measurement in anaesthesiology leads to better patient care. But not only that. By taking measurements, we acquire a better insight into what actually occurres during anaesthesia. In this way our knowledge is increased – knowledge which we will use for the benefit of our patients, present and future. Before we begin measuring, it is worthwhile to remember the 6 W's:

What   phenomena should we measure
Why   should we measure these phenomena
Which   methods should we use
Who   is responsible – legally and ethically
When   should we expect complications
Will   the equipment function correctly.

REFERENCES

1. Grabow, L., Sachs, W., Relinka, L., Schlemmer, H. & Ehekalt, V., Leistungs-psychologische und blutanalytische Untersuchungen bei Neuroleptanalgesien und Halothanenarkosen. *Anaesthesist* 22, 150 (1973).
2. Nunn, J. F., Oxygen. In: *Applied respiratory physiology.* p. 326. London 1969.
3. Nunn, J. F., Transport of oxygen to the brain. *Acta Anaesth. Scand.* Suppl. 45, 71 (1971).
4. Siesjö, B. K. & Plum, F., Cerebral energy metabolism in normoxia and hypoxia. *Acta Anaesth. Scand.* Suppl. 40, 81 (1971).
5. Huckabee, W. E., Relationship of pyruvate and lactate during anaerobic metabolism. *J. Clin. Invest.* 37, 244 (1958).
6. Clark, D. L. & Rosner, B. S., Neurophysiologic effects of general anesthetics:

I. The electroencephalogram and sensory evoked responses in man. *Anesthesiology* 38, 564 (1973).

7. Snow, J., Narcotism by the inhalation of vapors. The First Seven Parts, from the *London Medical Gazette*. London, Wilson and Ogilvy, 57 Skinner St., Snowhill 1848.

8. Eger, E. I., Saidman, L. J., Brandstater, B., et al., Minimum alveolar anesthetic concentration: A standard of anesthetic potency. *Anesthesiology* 26, 756-763 (1965).

9. Clark, D. L. & Rosner, B. S., Neurophysiologic effects of general anesthetics: II. Regional neural actions of anesthetics. *Anesthesiology* 39, 59 (1973).

10. Howat, D. D. C., Barker, J., Vale, R. J. G. & Ellis, F. R., Temperature regulation. *Anaesthesia* 28, 236-252 (1973).

11. Bossers, P. A., De beoordeling van reinheid en comfort in operatiekamers. In: *Klimaat installaties ziekenhuizen*. nr. publ. 434 IG – TNO Delft 1972.

12. Vale, R. J., Normothermia: its place in operative and post-operative care. *Anaesthesia* 28, 241 (1973).

13. Hekman, W. & Spierdijk, J., Thermoregulatie, belemmerd door shock en dehydratie. *Ned. T. Geneesk.* 106, 967 (1962).

14. Ellis, F. R., Malignant hyperpyrexia. *Anaesthesia* 28, 245 (1972).

15. Innes, R. K. & Strömme, J. K., Rise in serum creatine phosphokinase associated with agents used in anaesthesia. *Brit. J. Anaesth.* 45, 185 (1973).

16. Sayer, B. McA., The computer and the clinical sign. *Proc. Roy Soc. Med.* 66, 473 (1973).

17. Downs, J. B. et al., Hazards of radial-artery catheterization. *Anesthesiology* 38, 283 (1973).

18. Bedford, R. F. & Wollman, H. W., Complications of percutaneous radial-artery cannulation. *Anesthesiology* 38, 228 (1973).

19. Mathieu, A. et al., Expanding aneurysm of the radial-artery after frequent puncture. *Anesthesiology* 38, 401 (1973).

20. Barber, J. D., Wright, D. J. & Ellis, R. H., Radial artery puncture. A simple screening test of the ulnar anastomotic circulation. *Anaesthesia* 28, 291-293 (1973).

PROBLEMS OF INTERFERENCE AND ELECTRICAL SAFETY ASSOCIATED WITH RECORDING OF BIOLOGICAL SIGNALS

J. P. BLACKBURN

Electrical connections to the patient are made in many ways and for a variety of purposes. Electrodes are used for recording the electrocardiogram (ECG) and electroencephalogram (EEG) and other connections may be made via the diathermy, intracardiac pacemaker electrodes or a saline filled catheter. In addition, temperature sensors, flowmeters and other devices may be attached to the patient and he may also make electrical contact with conductors such as the bed frame, lamp or call system. Any of these connections may cause electrical interference on ECG or EEG recordings and under some circumstances there may be a danger of electrocution.

The most usual type of electrical interference arises form the alternating current (a.c.) mains supply, or from equipment connected to it, so it is worth considering first the mains supply normally provided at socket outlets and light fittings (1). This consists of:

a. A 'live' wire (L) which alternates at approximately 240 V 50 Hz with respect to local 'earth'.

b. A 'neutral' wire (N) carrying the return load current and which is near earth potential.

c. An 'earth' wire (E), not always present, which should be at local earth potential. This earth wire provides a return path for 'leakage currents' which always arise in equipment because of electrical pathways which exist between live and earthed parts of the instrument. In addition, the earth wire is usually connected to the case of the equipment and will protect the user if, under fault conditions, some live part of the device comes in contact with the case. Under these circumstances the earth wire will carry a large current and the equipment will remain near earth potential. If the fault current is large enough the fuse or circuit breaker will operate.

13

TYPES OF ELECTRICAL INTERFERENCE

Mains frequency interference, 'mains hum', may be troublesome during ECG or EEG recording, particularly when mains operated equipment is in use, such as in an operating theatre or intensive therapy unit. Unlike leads, amplifiers and recorders which can be 'screened' from some forms of interference, patients are physically large unscreened conductors and other techniques have to be used to reduce electrical interference.

i) Capacitively coupled interference.

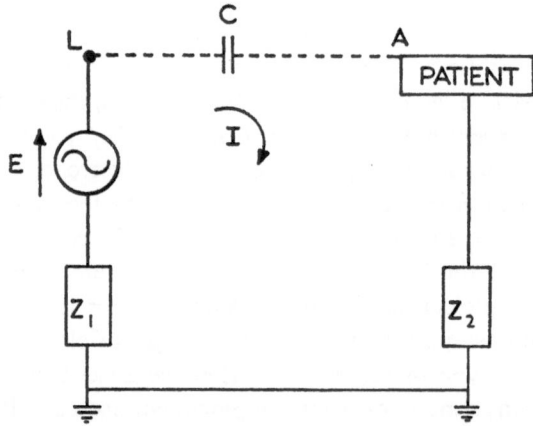

Fig. 1. Diagram showing electrical interference produced by capacitative coupling. L is the source of interference produced by the generator E. C is the imaginary capacitor linking the source of interference and the patient.

Interference is produced because of capacitative coupling between the source of interference and the patient, as shown in Fig. 1. The mains live conductor L acts as one plate of the capacitor C, while the patient is the other plate. The neutral side of the mains is connected to earth through an impedance Z_1 which usually has a low value. The patient is also connected to earth through the impedance Z_2. The size of Z_2 will depend very much on local conditions. It will be large if the patient is isolated from earth (for instance lying in bed) or may be very low if the patient is connected to earth (for instance by an earthed diathermy plate). When L goes positive with respect to earth, negative charges will be attracted towards the surface A and positive ones repelled. When E reverses in polarity, negative charges will be repelled at A and positive ones attracted. Thus a mains frequency current I flows through the patient, even though there is no direct electrical connection between the patient and the mains. Interference of this type can also be picked up by signal leads and electrical components in the amplifier.

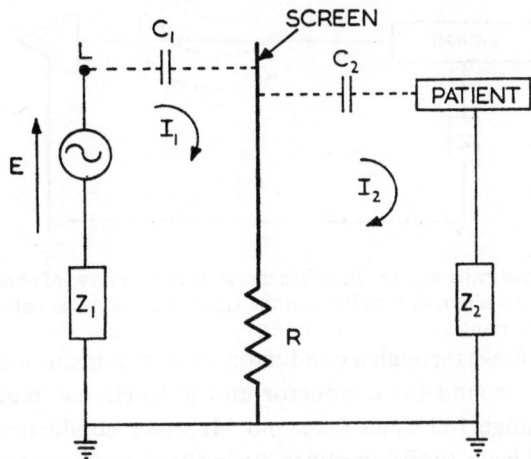

Fig. 2. A screen is used to reduce capacitively coupled interference. The screen is connected to the earth reference by a low resistance pathway R. The screen is coupled to the patient by C_2, but very little electrical interference is picked up because the screen is virtually at earth potential.

Capacitively coupled interference can be reduced by moving the patient away from the source of interference and by screening as much of the equipment as possible. The screen is a conductor connected by a low resistance pathway to earth placed between the source of interference and the patient and associated equipment, as shown in Fig. 2. C_1 and C_2 represent the capacitance between L and the screen and between screen and patient. R represents the low resistance of the screen and the wire connecting it to earth. A current I_1 flows from the source through the screen and there will thus be a potential difference across resistance R. As far as the patient is concerned this small potential difference across the screen now becomes the source of interference instead of E and consequently the lower R is made the less interference reaches the patient.

The screen can be a thin sheet of metal foil, a metal box or a wire mesh when flexibility is necessary, as with screened cables. Sources of interference should be screened as far as possible and so should signal leads and amplifiers.

ii) Electromagnetically induced interference.

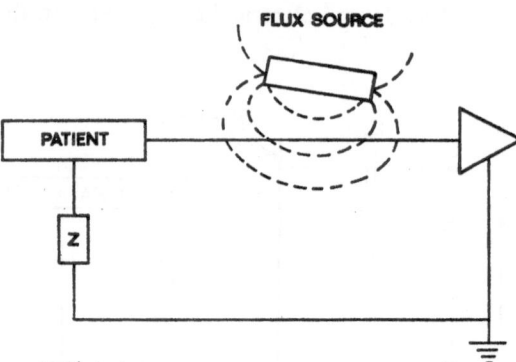

Fig. 3. Electromagnetically induced interference, showing a source of alternating magnetic flux which induces an alternating voltage in the signal lead between patient and amplifier (represented by the triangle).

When a current flows through a conductor, such as a mains lead, it generates a magnetic flux around the conductor and if 50 Hz a.c. mains is flowing, the flux will change 100 times a second. If other conductors, such as the patient or signal leads to the amplifier, lie in the changing magnetic flux then voltages will be induced in the conductors. A simple circuit is shown in Fig. 3, where hum is induced in the signal lead to the amplifier. This effect is similar to that used in a transformer and electromagnetically induced interference can be reduced by making the transformer as inefficient as possible. Sources of interference should be kept as far away from the patient and associated equipment as possible and the signal leads should be kept close together. Twisting the leads also helps to cancel out induced voltages. It is usually impossible to screen the source of interference, as large amounts of soft iron would have to be used to confine the lines of flux.

In spite of screening and other precautions it is likely that the patient will be subjected to electrical interference which may be many times larger than the ECG signal which is being recorded. A simple 'single ended' amplifier such as that shown in Fig. 3, where there is one active input and the circuit is completed by an earth reference serving both the patient and the amplifier, will be inadequate unless signal levels are one volt or more. For recording small signals such as the ECG a more complex 'differential input' amplifier must be used. This has two active inputs symmetrically arranged with respect to the reference (usually earth) and operates as follows: signals appearing between the two inputs are amplified, while signals which affect the two inputs equally with respect to the earth reference are not amplified. Electrical changes affecting both inputs equally are said to be 'in-phase' and the in-phase rejection of an amplifier may be 10,000:1. This means that for a given change in the output, the signal affecting both inputs equally would need to be 10,000 times larger than a signal applied between the two active inputs. This technique is used to reduce a potent cause of electrical interference, because mains hum affecting both inputs equally with respect to earth will not appear at the output.

iii) Earth loops.

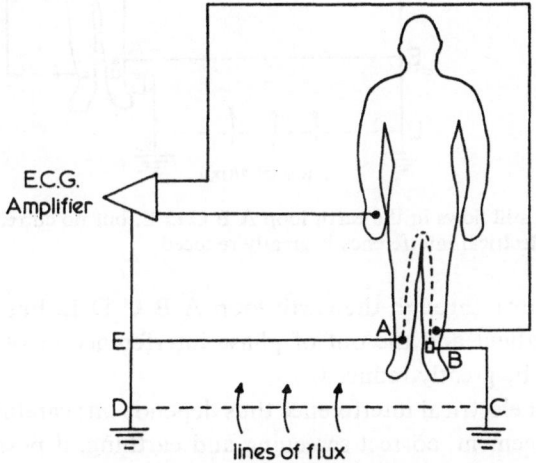

Fig. 4. Two earth connections are made on the patient (A and B). A current flows through the earth loop A B C D E which includes the patient, as a result of electromagnetic coupling.

Hum can also be induced in the earth wiring as shown in Fig. 4. The patient's right leg is connected to mains earth reference by an ECG machine and the left leg is connected to earth via a diathermy plate. Lead II of the ECG is recorded using a differential input amplifier. An earth loop A B C D E has been produced and as part of the earth wiring lies alongside mains power cables it is inevitable that the earth conductors will be cut by changing electromagnetic flux and consequently a current will flow in the earth loop. This mains frequency current flows through the patient, shown diagrammatically by the dotted line, and it is highly unlikely that it will affect both the signal electrodes equally. Thus mains hum will be amplified and displayed together with the ECG signal.

If, on the other hand, the earthed diathermy plate is connected to the patient's right leg, as shown in Fig. 5, the situation is improved considerably.

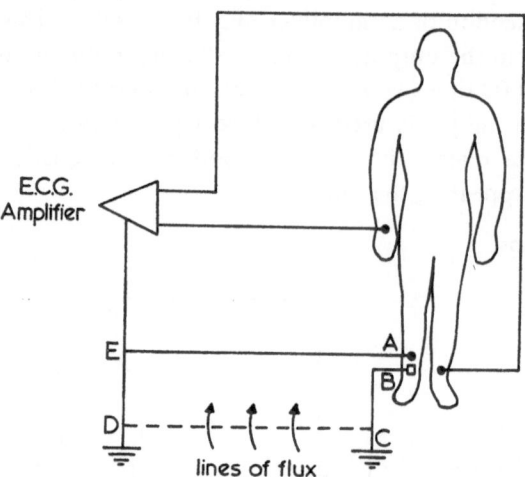

Fig. 5. A current still flows in the earth loop A B C D E, but no current passes through the patient and electrical interference is greatly reduced.

Current still flows through the earth loop A B C D E, but this no longer involves the patient and the out of phase interference involving the signal electrodes will be greatly reduced.

Reduction of electrical interference thus depends on: careful electrode and signal lead placement, correct screening and earthing, if possible with only one earth point on the patient, and well designed equipment (high in-phase rejection ratio).

ELECTRICAL SAFETY

The possibility of electrocution increases as more and more electrical equipment is used at the bedside and it is important that doctors and nurses are aware of the hazards and that the equipment is regularly serviced.

(i) Electric shock.

If electrodes are placed on the surface of the body and a voltage applied between them, then a current will flow depending on the impedance of the pathway. The resistance (or more correctly the impedance) involved is very variable, the resistance between the surface of the skin and the underlying tissues varies between several million ohms and tens of thousands of ohms depending on local conditions. If electrode jelly is used to reduce skin resistance, it usually falls to about one thousand ohms but may be as low as 300 ohms.

When surface electrodes are applied to the limbs only a small fraction of the current flows through the heart because of the multiplicity of available pathways and in general if 50 Hz a.c. is used the following effects are found:

Threshold of feeling	0.5	– 2 mA
Muscular paralysis	25	– 100 mA
Ventricular fibrillation	30	– 200 mA (typically 70 mA)

The frequency of the stimulating current is important. If direct current is used, about five times the current is required, while large high frequency currents pass through the body without ill effect when the diathermy is used.

Provided the electrical installation and the equipment are well maintained then direct electrocution of the patient is very rare and usually at least two faults have to be present before the patient is at risk. Earthing the equipment protects the user from leakage currents which normally exist, as previously mentioned, and ensures that metal parts of the instrument remain at earth potential should a fault develop. In addition, the earth connection reduces capacitively coupled electrical interference.

The commonest electrical fault in mains operated equipment is disconnection of the earth wire. Usually the device will operate apparently normally in this condition so that the user is unaware that a potentially hazardous situation exists. If, however, a second fault now develops the case or other parts of the instrument may become 'live' and cause electrocution.

Small potential differences are likely to exist between the power supply neutral and local earth and even between local earth connections in different parts of the building. The importance of these small voltage differences will be considered below.

(ii) Microelectrocution.

Very small currents may produce ventricular fibrillation when intracardiac electrodes are used or when a saline filled catheter provides a conducting pathway within the heart, as all the current flows across the myocardium. A small electrode in contact with ventricular muscle is most likely to produce ventricular fibrillation and a current of 180 μA has been reported by Whalen et al. (2) to produce ventricular fibrillation in man. Usually much larger currents are required, however, and about 1 mA is needed to produce ventricular fibrillation with the electrode in the ventricle, while ventricular fibrillation cannot be produced with currents of up to 10 mA using an atrial electrode in dogs (3). Small currents, which can endanger the patient, are found even when equipment is working normally and may be difficult to detect. The possibility of microelectrocution should always be considered when there is a catheter or other electrical connection in the ventricle, particularly if dysrhythmias occur in association with gross electrical interference on the ECG.

Differences in potential may be found between earth terminals even in the same room and if leads from equipment earthed some distance away (for instance at a central monitoring station) are applied to a patient, together with locally earthed devices then there may be a difference of several volts between the two earth points. Thus, not only will there be large earth loops which are likely to cause interference, but also the patient may be in danger of microelectrocution.

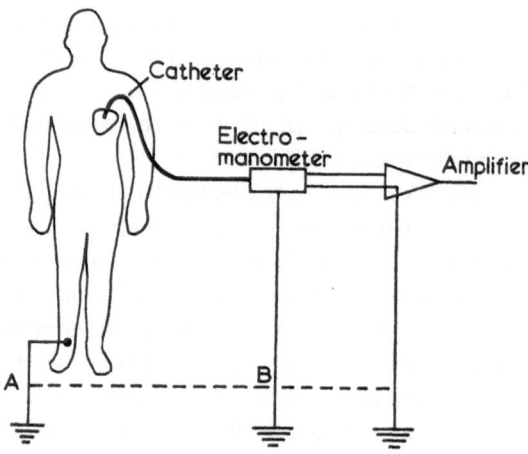

Fig. 6. The patient and equipment are earthed at A and B. If these points are at different potentials then current will flow across the myocardium.

The situation in shown diagramatically in Fig. 6, where the patient is earthed through the right leg lead of an ECG machine at A and via a saline filled electromanometer (B) and amplifier. If these earths are at different potentials then a current will flow across the myocardium. The situation is improved both with regard to electrical interference and patient safety if the equipment is all plugged into a single group of power sockets sharing a common earth so that A and B are at the same potential. If necessary, other metal objects within reach of the patient should also be connected to this common earth point. This ensures that all contacts made to the patient, either deliberate or accidental, are at the same potential and no current can flow through the patient.

When the patient must be earthed, there should only be a single earth connection if possible, to avoid the problems of earth loops discussed above. Ideally the patient should be isolated from earth whenever possible (4, 5).

Isolated pacemakers are used routinely and isolated ECG machines and electromanometers are now available. These may be battery driven, or special circuitry involving transformer or optical coupling may isolate the patient leads from mains earth. Equipment is available where the leakage current to earth is less than 10 μA under the worst conditions. Dobbie (6) considers this specification unnecessarily stringent, but points out (7), that monitoring equipment supplied from a low voltage transformer will not only cause less electrical interference but will also be safe and have a low leakage current without the need for elaborate circuitry.

If patient monitoring and other equipment is to be safe it must be efficiently maintained. As previously mentioned, the commonest fault is disconnection of the earth lead, which many often pass unnoticed unless the equipment is checked regularly.

Now that the introduction of conducting devices within the heart has become relatively commonplace, it has become easy to produce ventricular fibrillation in patients with currents of only a few hundred microamps which are likely to be undetected. Small currents can flow across the myocardium both when the equipment appears to be operating normally, as well as under fault conditions. It is important that manufacturers and users of electromedical equipment are aware of these hazards and are able to avoid them in practice.

REFERENCES

1. Dobbie, A. K., Electricity in hospitals. *Biomed. Engng.* 7, 12 (1972).
2. Whalen, R. E., Starmer, C. F. & McIntosh, H. D., Electrical hazards associated with cardiac pacemaking. *Ann. N.Y. Acad. Sci.* 111, 922 (1964).
3. Green, H. L., Raftery, E. B. & Gregory, I. C., Ventricular fibrillation threshold of healthy dogs to 50 Hz current in relation to earth leakage currents of electromedical equipment. *Biomed. Engng.* 7, 408 (1972).
4. Pocock, S. N., Part 1: Principles, practice and hazards: Earth-free patient monitoring. *Biomed. Engng.* 7, 21 (1972).
5. Pocock, S. N., Part 2: Design and specification: Earth-free patient monitoring. *Biomed. Engng.* 7, 67 (1972).
6. Dobbie, A. K., Is money for safety unlimited? *Biomed. Engng.* 10, 542 (1972).
7. Dobbie, A. K., Patient safety – class III equipment has advantages. *Biomed. Engng.* 8, 20 (1973).

THE SCOPE OF MEASUREMENTS USING RADIOACTIVE ISOTOPES

K. STEINBEREITHNER

INTRODUCTION

Even though nuclear medicine has developed a variety of methods which are of interest to us, the use of radioactive isotopes for measurements before, during and after clinical anaesthesia, in anaesthesiological research, and in the field of intensive care is still relatively limited despite several research findings of extraordinary significance. This remains true despite constantly increasing automation which has enabled faster acquisition of important data.

The reasons why we largely dispense with these important aids are not easy to analyze. Besides the 'innate' shyness of medical experts with regard to technological developments, a 'closed-shop' way of thinking, characterizing isotope experts undoubtedly plays a certain role. In addition, many physicians are scared of the great amount of time and equipment required. This is even more complicated by the fact that certain examinations require the patient to be taken to the bulky equipment and not vice versa (e.g. scanning or examinations with a gamma- (Anger-) camera). As our own experience has shown, this frequently involves great organizational difficulties. Furthermore, some of the techniques are comparatively unreliable in more severe pathological conditions. Alternatively, they may be so complex and time-consuming that they cannot be applied to very sick patients to obtain initial data before starting therapy (e.g. patients in shock). (The aspect of exposure to radiation, however, can be left out of consideration even in case of repeated measurements).

There is one further factor: the lack of awareness of most investigators of many of these possibilities. This seems to increase rather than decrease as a result of insufficient communication between our specialty and nuclear medicine experts. Unfortunately, this applies also to the author of this paper, who has experiences in a few fields only and has therefore to resort to the appropriate literature in other fields.

CHARACTERISTICS OF A TRACER

Before going into details, it might be useful to recall briefly the properties of a radioactive tracer to be used in compartment analyses and examinations of excretion and/or metabolism (1, 2, 3). They are in particular:

a. Use in harmless dosage without untoward side-effects in a small volume (no disturbance or the steady state).

b. Limitation to the compartment to be measured over a sufficiently long period of time (see below).

c. Labelled as well as unlabelled substances should undergo the same metabolic changes.

d. Stable tracer binding (no exchange, no splitting).

The requirement listed under d. is frequently not met. This has been demonstrated, for example, by Swan and Nelson (4) during investigations carried out with commercially available ^{125} RIHSA, cf. Fig. 1.

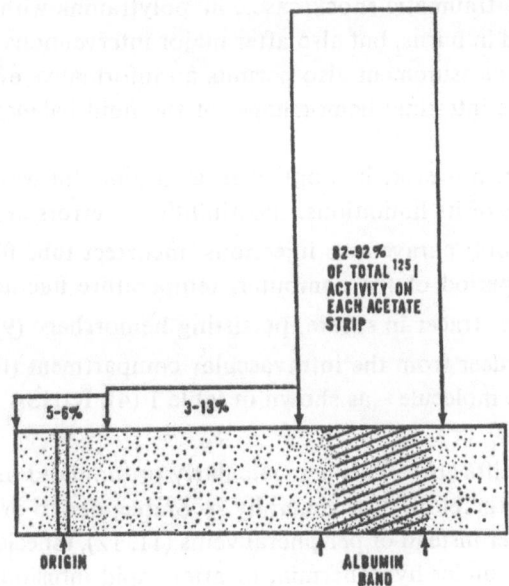

Fig. 1. Electrophoresis of ^{125}RIHSA (schematic graph) 8-18% of radioactivity outside the albumin-band (from (4)).

MEASUREMENT OF BLOOD VOLUME (BV)

The use of radioactive substances for BV measurements is on the basis of dilution. Determination of the ratio total amount of tracer/final concentration in blood according to the formula

$$BV = \frac{C_1 \times \text{volume of tracer}}{C_2}$$

has become a widely applied method (5), when C_1 and C_2 are respectively the initial and final concentration of the tracer. With the use of computers, measurements are rather speedy to accomplish and can (with certain restrictions) be repeated several times (6). The indicators used are labelled albumin – [131] RIHSA, [125] RIHSA. The latter is preferred nowadays because of its longer half-life. Erythrocytes tagged with ^{51}Cr may also be employed. A great number of measuring devices used with direct volume indication and digital memories are available for repeated measurements (e.g. Volemetron/Ames; Hemolitre/Picker; Blood Volume Computer/Pitman).

CLINICAL OBSERVATIONS

The repeated measurement of blood volume is a valuable aid, not only for the treatment of traumatic shock cases, in polytrauma without any visible hemorrhage, and in burns, but also after major interventions such as cardiac operations. BV measurement also permits an informative evaluation of the progress of acute intestinal hemorrhage, of the fluid balance in peritonitis, anuria, etc. (7).

The method can, however, be applied in a meaningful way only if one is constantly aware of its limitations. Possibilities of errors are:

a. Technical errors: paravenous injections, incorrect tube filling, too short warming-up period of the computer, temperature fluctuations, etc. (8).

b. Dilution of the tracer in severe, persisting hemorrhage (9).

c. Loss of the tracer from the intravascular compartment (this depends on the size of the molecule – as shown in table 1 (4), RIHSA permeates with particular ease).

d. Hematocrit shifts (10). This is particularly pronounced in venous engorgement. It is therefore now generally recommended to draw blood from a caval catheter instead of peripheral veins (11, 12), especially if vasopressors are used, under hypothermia, or after rapid infusions, etc. (10).

e. Insufficient time allowed for mixing, expecially in cases of severe shock, when plasma tracers achieve an equilibrium after a maximum time of 20 minutes (13) and ^{51}Cr, only after one hour or more (14).

The quarrel between two 'hostile camps' as to which method (RIHSA or chromiumtagged erythrocytes) can be regarded as really reliable, has considerably subsided. Undoubtedly, both methods have their disadvantages. With the ^{51}Cr method it is particularly the increased amount of time required for mixing. There are various 'simultaneous' methods but this approach does not offer clinical advantages despite additional 'memory display units' (15).

Table 1. Capillary wall permeation of tracers

SWAN and NELSON 1971 (4)
T-1824 or ^{131}I-albumin > dextrane (200.000) >
^{131}I-globulin > ^{131}I-fibrinogen > ^{51}Cr-RBC

Rustad (13) and Ladegaard–Pedersen (16) made the very fruitful suggestions to compensate the different measuring values obtained by the two methods (with ^{51}Cr about 10% too low, with RIHSA about 9% too high) (13), which leads to the well-known total difference of 15-20% (4, 9) by applying appropriate correction factors. These correction factors are summarized in table 2.

Table 2. Correction factors in BV-estimations

RUSTAD (13), ALBERT (3) and LADEGAARD–PEDERSEN (16)

LHV (large vessel hematocrit) × 0,95 (0,96-0,97):
Trapped plasma

LHV × 0,9 (0,91): whole body hematocrit (WBH)

BV (RIHSA) × $\dfrac{100 - WBH}{100 - 0,9 \times WBH}$ ($\approx$ 0,94):
Correction for overestimation

BV (^{51}Cr) × $\dfrac{1}{0,9}$ ($\approx$1,1): correction for underestimation (WBH)

RCV (red cell volume) × 0,9 (= BV_{CORR} × Hct_{CORR} × 0,9):
WBH-correction

PV_d (plasma volume derived) = BV_{CORR} - RCV_{CORR}

Although RIHSA-BV correction as well as RCV (red cell volume) correction appear somewhat empirical, their use leads, as our own experience has shown, to an excellent correspondence, for instance, between calculated and measured plasma volume values (see table 3). As indicated in Fig. 2, this

Table 3. Influence of correction factors on PV estimations (correlation: BV-derivation vs. direct measurement in 2 series of experiments evaluating plasma expanders)

	N	r	significance
preinfusion (uncorr.)	14	0,72	< 0,01
preinfusion (corr.)		0,93	< 0,001
postinfusion (uncorr.)	13	0,21	> 0,1
postinfusion (corr.)		0,88	< 0,001

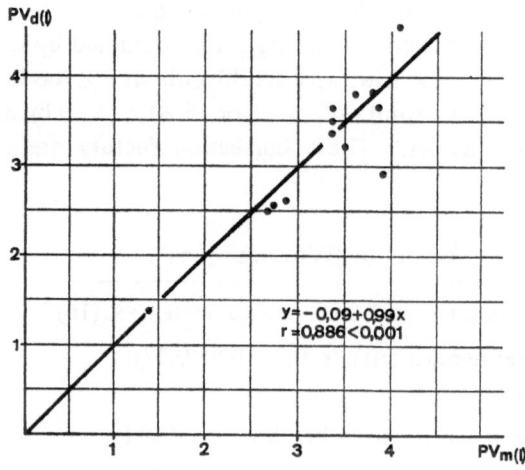

Fig. 2. Correlation: directly measured PV_m vs. 'derived' PV_d using appropriate correction factors ([131] RIHSA-method/Volemetron; estimation immediately after rapid infusion of 1000 ml expander solution).

applies also to measurements performed after a rapid infusion (1,000 ml in one hour), although in this case one would expect a wider range of error (10). Regardless of the pitfalls just discussed, we can hardly do without a blood volume computer in operating theatres and intensive care units. However, the blood volume should always be correlated with other parameters (indirect indicators), as e.g. red blood count, hematocrit, central venous pressure, and urine volume per hour. The opinion of several authors, saying that the measurement of the central venous pressure could replace BV measurement cannot be shared by us. As shown in Fig. 3 (17), there is a far-reaching synchronization between CVP and BV, but the variations of the measuring values are much too great to allow binding conclusions to be

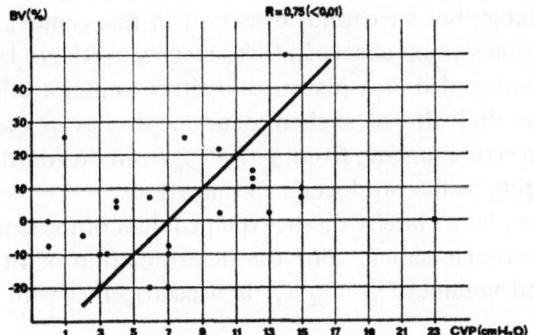

Fig. 3. Correlation: BV vs. CVP in chronically infused intensive care patients. R = Spearman's rank correlation coefficient. Regression line drawn arbitrarily (from (17)).

drawn from one measuring parameter. A special warning seems to be indicated with regard to the sole use of ^{51}Cr in severe cases of hemorrhage. As shown in Fig. 4 (after 9), the tracer dilution with a respective pseudo-increase of the BV can lead to completely erroneous conclusions.

Finally, some remarks concerning the possible applications of the BV computer for other types of investigations:

1. Examination of the effect of blood substitutes; comprehensive literature

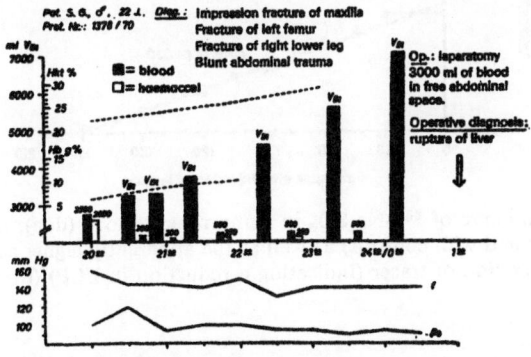

Fig. 4. Results of successive BV-determinations with ^{51}Cr in a trauma case with severe intraabdominal bleeding. Fictitious BV-increase caused by continuous tracer loss (from (9)).

on that is available, but we cannot discuss it in this context. Presently, we are investigating the volume effect of a 1,8⁰/₀ Dextrane-Ringer-lactate solution, which was recommended as a plasma substitute amongst others by Gollub et al. (18). The difficulty of such measurements lies in the fact that the method leads to errors ranging from ± 7-12 % from the fourth measurement onward, according to the producer's specifications.

In this context, let us briefly discuss the problem of the extracellular fluid (ECF) in hemorrhagic shock. For the determination of ECF (Which includes the blood volume) $^{35}S-Na_2SO_4$ is used together with blood volume tracers (19).

Unlike Shires (20), who observed an extreme reduction of ECF in patients in shock and from this concluded that infusion therapy with Ringer's lactate was indicated, various subsequent researchers (19, 21, 22) have not found any discordant behaviour of ECF and BV. This may have been partly the result of the inherent errors in the method (different mixing time; reduced ^{35}S excretion in shock), leading to an apparent ECF reduction (21), cf. Fig. 5.

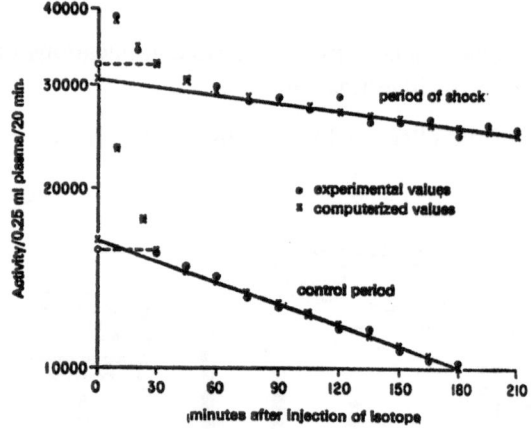

Fig. 5. Equilibrium curve of $^{35}S-Na_2SO_2$ in hemorrhagic shock (dog); note the delayed mixing time (compared with controls) as well as the apparently higher activity caused by decreased renal excretion of tracer (indicating a reduction in ECF) (from (21)).

2. Determination of the disappearance rate as a parameter of capillary permeability. As already mentioned, after a certain period of time RIHSA leaves the vascular system, the rate depending on the permeability of the

capillaries (2). From the decrease of activity we can calculate the 1 hour disappearance rate (after extrapolation) by the equation

$$\frac{BV_{60} - BV_0}{BV_{60}} \times 100 \quad (23).$$

Fig. 6 shows the results of such an examination carried out by the author. These show that the plasma disappearance rate is normally about 9%/hour. After surgery of the epigastric region it rises to almost 19%, whereas 24 hours oxygen therapy significantly ($p < 0,01$) reduces the disappearance rate to 13%. The observed disappearence rates after surgery are extraordinarily high if compared with those described by Rustad (13), and their extent may be compared only with the protein loss in burns. They correspond, however, to values we have obtained by using other methods. The favourable effect of post-operative oxygen therapy in this respect has not been described by others yet, as far as we know.

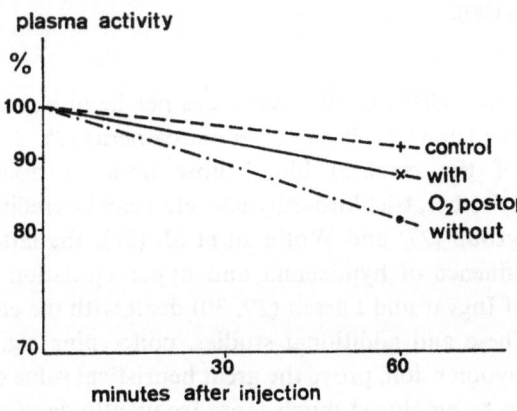

Fig. 6. Plasma disappearance rates of ¹³¹RIHSA after abdominal operations with and without postoperative oxygen application via nasal catheter (oxygen vs. no oxygen $p < 0,01$) (from (23)).

MEASUREMENT OF ORGAN BLOOD FLOW

1. *Brain.* Among the numerous organs which permit the use of isotopes for perfusion measurements the brain has been most intensively investigated in a systematic manner. A number of isotopes were tested for their applicability, e.g. ⁹⁹ᵐTc, ⁸⁵Kr, ⁸⁵ᵐKr, ¹³³Xe, as well as recently also ¹⁵O (in order to determine O_2-consumption simultaneously). Among all these methods (survey in 24), only ⁸⁵Kr- and ¹³³Xe-clearance have achieved real clinical value, particularly since not only total blood flow, but also the regional

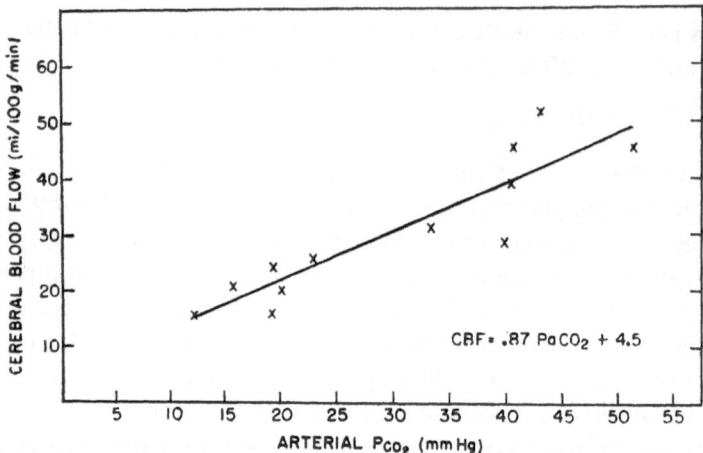

Fig. 7. Cerebral blood flow as a function of arterial PCO_2 during anaesthesia (thiopentone-N_2O-d-tubocurarine): decrease to 1/3 of normal after vigorous hyperventilation (^{85}Kr-method; from (28)).

cerebral blood flow (rCBF) in 50 - 100 areas per hemisphere can be determined with multi-channel analyzers (gamma camera) (25, 26).

Measurements of the cerebral blood flow under various anaesthetics (halothane, diethyl-ether, trichloro-ethylene, etc.) can be credited particularly to McDowall's group (27) and Wollman et al. (28), the latter having also examined the influence of hypoxemia and hyperventilation (Fig. 7). The Swedish group of Ingvar and Lassen (29, 30) dealt with the effects of neuroleptanalgesia. These and additional studies, concerning e.g. the effects of vasopressors or hypotension, prove the great heuristical value of this method, which deserves to be employed much more frequently despite the organizational difficulties mentioned before. One example taken from the field of intensive care which was studied by our group (26) shall be given a more detailed discussion:

In the chronically persistent apallic syndrome after cranio-cerebral traumata it is extraordinarily difficult to make any conclusive statement on its prognosis; therefore we measure, as part of our routine work, the rCBF if signs of remittance are absent after 6-8 weeks. If the rCBF in the majority of areas falls below the standard by more than 50% (Fig. 8) – accompanied usually by a shift in perfusion ratio in favour of the white matter – and if confirmed by EEG, pneumoencephalography findings, etc. (31), we terminate the 'intensive care' regime in favour of 'normal' therapy.

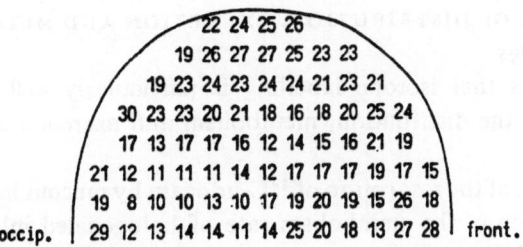

```
                    22 24 25 26
                19 26 27 27 25 23 23
             19 23 24 23 24 24 21 23 21
          30 23 23 20 21 18 16 18 20 25 24
          17 13 17 17 16 12 14 15 16 21 19
       21 12 11 11 11 14 12 17 17 17 19 17 15
       19  8 10 10 13 10 17 19 20 19 15 26 18
occip. 29 12 13 14 14 11 14 25 20 18 13 27 28  front.
```

Fig. 8. rCBF (right hemisphere) on 66th day after severe brain trauma in a case of apallic syndrome; note the extremely low temporal and occipital rCBF areas (overall hemispheric flow 21,8 ml/100 g/min) (from (26)).

2. *Other organs.* Blood flow measurements in other organs, e.g. *liver*, *kidney* (including functional scintigraphy) do not have any practical significance for the work of the anaesthetist, since their value in yielding accurate data is still highly disputed (Isotope nephrography performed for a short time at our intensive care unit in kidney transplantations was not very successful). *Pulmonary scintigraphy* will be dealt with later. Holzman et al. (32) suggest a method which might be of interest in estimating the effects of conductive anaesthesia (nerve blocks) by measuring *muscular blood flow*. Although it actually represents a dilution technique, we would like to refer to a very elegant method for 'precordial' determination of *cardiac output* with ^{131}RIHSA (33), which, combined with BV measurements, permits serial tests (Fig. 9 shows such a radiograph with evaluated results); the results achieved by this method correspond excellently to those obtained using the Fick principle.

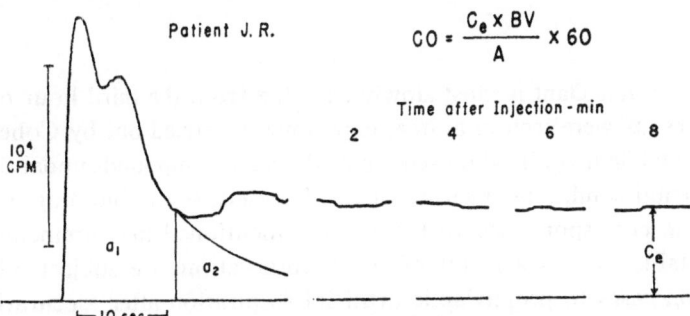

$$CO = \frac{C_e \times BV}{A} \times 60$$

Fig. 9. Precordial cardiac output (CO) determination with ^{131}RIHSA (injection via superior vena cava catheter). C_e:equilibrium concentration; A:curve areas ($a_1 + a_2$); BV:blood volume (from (33)).

EXAMINATION OF DISTRIBUTION, EXCRETION AND METABOLISM

1. *Labelled drugs*

a. It is obvious that isotope labelling is particularly well suited for the examination of the distribution, metabolism and excretion of anaesthetics. Examples are:

1. Examination of the resorption of ^{14}C-lidocain by mucous membranes (34).
2. Determination of the metabolism rate of halogenated inhalation anaesthetics, e.g. ^{14}C-halothane (35).

b. Of at least the same clinical value are investigations concerning the fate of relaxants. Fig. 10 (36) shows the results of our own examinations regarding plasma activity of ^{3}H-diallyl-nor-toxiferine (Dant) in kidney transplantations.

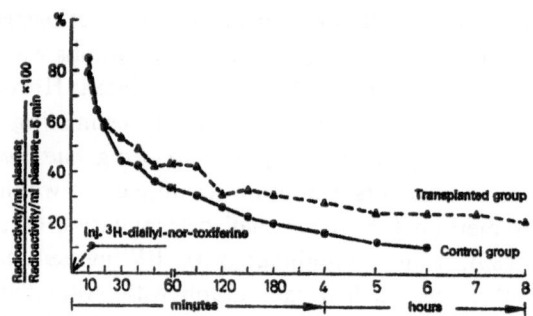

Fig. 10. Plasma activity of ^{3}H-diallyl-nor-toxiferine (% of 5 min. value) in kidney transplant cases (from (36)).

They prove that Dant is most slowly excreted from the third hour onward; similar results were seen in animal experiments carried out by Cohen et al. (37) and Dal Santo (38), who used labelled curare compounds under different experimental conditions (ligature of renal vessels, severe bleeding, hypoxia, etc.). The correspondence with the abovementioned measurements is excellent (table 4). As a result of these observations we subject all transplantation cases to prophylactic artificial respiration after 'decurarization' for a period of 8-12 hours (39). Renal (and hepatic) excretion of *all* relaxants which are not metabolized should be principally examined in this way in order to avoid severe incidents (cf. 36).

Table 4. Decrease of plasma activity in %(5 min-value = 100%)

time after injection (min)	COHEN (dTC) (37)		own results (DANT)	
	controls	ligature renal vessels	controls	transplant cases
15	—	—	64	64
30	—	—	44	53
60	27	30	33	43
120	17	27	26	31
180	10	24	19	31

2. Compartment analysis
a. Investigations related to the distribution of ^{35}S-Na$_2$SO$_4$ in the ECF compartment have already been discussed.
b. A method, suggested by Chinard and Enns (40) as early as 1954, has recently achieved serious attention: the measurement of transcapillary exchange of water and/or 'extravascular lung water'. By determining the differences between the distribution compartments of two tracers (^{131}RIHSA on the one hand and ^{3}H$_2$0 or ^{131}I-antipyrin (41) on the other), a more profound knowledge of intrapulmonary water shifts in shock can be obtained (42), both after lung transplantations and in the so-called respirator lung syndrome. However, the clinical value of such examinations (possibly in combination with the measurement of the distribution of diffusible gases, as e.g. N$_2$0 or ^{15}0$_2$) has been commented on with some reservation (43).

3. Erythrocyte 'survival'
One example of the various possibilities of *hematological* examinations in the field of intensive therapy is the determination of the erythrocyte 'survival' (44). At our intensive care unit we have tried (45) to find out more about the reasons for anemia after cerebral trauma. We have found that this phenomenon is particularly pronounced in the second week of illness, and is closely related to an unexplained reduction of the survival time of red blood cells to approximately half of its usual value (table 5).

PULMONARY FUNCTION STUDIES
The advent of sequential scintigraphy with the gamma camera has made it

Table 5.

Mean erythrocyte survival (^{51}Cr-method) in 8 cases of cerebral trauma

patient	age	sex	days
1	42	M	17,5
2	17	M	20
3	25	M	12
4	46	M	7,5
5	40	F	19,5
6	45	M	8
7	22	M	16
8	37	M	9,5/23
			$\overline{\times}$ 15,8
	normal values	27	– 32

possible to observe regional pulmonary function. Gaseous ^{133}Xe is used for ventilation measurements and ^{99m}Tc macro-particles or dissolved ^{133}Xe for perfusion examinations. After processing of the respective activity data as a 'contour plot', indices of lung volume, perfusion and ventilation, and also $\dot{V}/\dot{Q}$ ratio can be determined (46, 47, 48 – Fig. 11).

In combination with both X-ray examinations and gas analysis, this procedure could be valuable in the evaluation of changes in the lung during prolonged respirator treatment. Technical considerations do limit systematical examinations in our field. However, Strieder et al. (49) showed, in dogs undergoing artificial ventilation following pulmonary transplantation, that these obstacles are not insurmountable.

These methods can also be used for other purposes, e.g. for testing nebulizers. In order to test the efficiency of a nebulizer in inhalation therapy (Bird-Assistor), we used ^{99m}Tc-sulfur-colloid. Only 5 per cent becomes active in the body – the remainder being deposited in the ventilator system or lost through the exhalation valve. Out of these 5 per cent 50 % pass to the stomach, the remainder arriving at the lung during normal respiration. During faulty upper thoracic breathing it was mainly deposited in the glottic region. This result largely corresponds to investigations done by West and Dollery (50) and Wolfsdorf and Swift (51) and detracts more than somewhat from the highly praised 'mist' therapy.

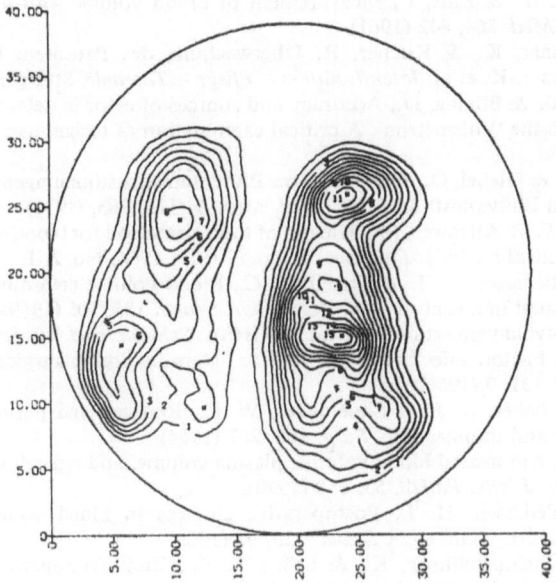

Fig. 11. Computer generated contour plot of ⁹⁹mTc-labelled serum albumin activity (lung perfusion) in a case of chronic obstructive lung disease (from (46)).

CONCLUDING REMARKS

This somewhat brief outline (deliberately neglecting radio-immuno-assay techniques) has shown that presently radioisotopes are used only in a most limited way in the practice of anaesthesia and its sub-specialties. Apart from exceptions such as BV measurement, there are only a few working groups who routinely employ methods offered by nuclear medicine. Considering the degree of applicability of these procedures, it would seem highly desirable that anaesthetists make more use of them. We hope that this paper gives some stimulus in this direction.

REFERENCES

1. Atkins, G. L., *Multicompartment Models for Biological Systems.* London 1969.
2. Albert, S. N., Blood Volume. Springfield 1963.
3. Albert, S. N., Blood volume. *Anesthesiology* 24, 231 (1963).
4. Swan, H. & Nelson, A. W., Blood volume I: Critique: Spun vs. isotope hematocrit; ¹²⁵ RIHSA vs. ⁵¹ CrRbC. *Ann.Surg.* 173, 481 (1971).
5. Freinkel, N., Schreiner, G. E. & Athens, J. W., Simultaneous distribution of T-1824 and I-131 labeled serum albumin in man. *J. clin. Invest.* 32, 138 (1953).

6. Williams, J. A. & Fine, J., Measurement of blood volume with a new apparatus. *N. Engl. J. Med.* 264, 842 (1961).
7. Steinbereithner, K. & Kucher, R. Überwachung des Patienten. In: Kucher, R., Steinbereithner, K. et al. *Intensivstation – Pflege – Therapie,* Stuttgart 1972.
8. Ulmer, H. V. & Böning, D., Accuracy and sources of error in determining the blood volume with the 'Volemetron'. A critical examination of techniques. *Anaesthesist* 20, 277 (1971).
9. Doehn, M. & Giebel, O., Der Wert von Blutvolumenbestimmungen bei akutem und chronischem Blutverlust. *Melsung. Med. Mitt.* 44/113, 283, (1970).
10. Gruber, U. F. & Allgöwer, M., The use of the volemetron for blood volume measurements. A critical analysis. *Bull. Soc. Internat. Chir.* 1964, No. 2, 1.
11. Ladegaard-Pedersen, H. J. & Engell, H. C., Blood volume determination using one catheter located in a central vein, *Acta. Chir. Scand.* 135, 105 (1969).
12. Lévy, J., Blutvolumenbestimmung mit R^{131}IHSA, *Schweiz. med. Wschr.* 100, 451 (1970).
13. Rustad, H., Factors affecting blood volume determination in surgical patients. *Acta Chir. Scand.* 131, 9 (1966).
14. Suzuki, F., Baker, R. J. & Shoemaker, W. C., Red cell and plasma volume after hemorrhage and trauma. *Ann. Surg.* 160, 263 (1964).
15. Free, A. H., Automated blood volume, plasma volume, and red cell volume measurements. *Amer. J. clin. Pathol.* 53, 688 (1970).
16. Ladegaard-Pedersen, H. J., Postoperative changes in blood volume and colloid osmotic pressure. *Acta. Chir. Scand.* 135, 95 (1969).
17. Mach, K., Steinbereithner, K. & Stöckelle, G., Zum Aussagewert des zentralen Venendruckes und anderer Meßgrößen des Flüssigkeitshaushaltes bei Intensivpatienten. *Wien. klin. Wschr.* 85, 639 (1973).
18. Gollub., S., Vanichanan, C., Schaefer, C. & Schechter, D. Ch., A study of safer plasma substitutes. *Surg. Gynec. Obstet.* 128, 1235 (1969).
19. Albert, S. N., Shibuya, J., Economopoulos, B., Radice, A., Cuevo, N., Varrone, E. V. & Albert, C. A., Simultaneous measurement of Erythrocyte, plasma and extracellular fluid volumes with radioactive tracers. *Anesthesiology* 29, 908 (1968).
20. Shires, T., Coln, D., Carrico, J. & Lightfoot, S., Fluid therapy in hemorrhagic shock. *Arch. Surg.,* 88, 688 (1964).
21. Roth, E., Lax, L. C. & Maloney, J. V., Veränderungen der extracellulären Flüssigkeit und des Blutvolumens im hämorrhagischen Schock. *Zschr. ges. exper. Med.* 147, 346 (1968).
22. Virtue, R. W., LeVine, D. S. & Aikawa, J. K., Fluid shifts during the surgical period: RISA and S^{35} determinations following glucose, saline or lactate infusion. *Ann. Surg.* 163, 523 (1966).
23. Böhmig, H. J., Fraundorfer, G. & Steinbereithner, K., Untersuchungen zur postoperativen Sauerstofftherapie: Die Plasmaverschwinderate von Radiojodalbumin unter dem Einfluß postoperativer Sauerstoffapplikation. *Wien. klin. Wschr.* 76, 172 (1964).
24. Brock, M., Fieschi, C., Ingvar, D. H., Lassen, N. A. & Schürmann, K. (ed.) *Cerebral Blood Flow.* Berlin 1969.
25. Ingvar, D. H. & Lassen, N. A., Regional blood flow of the cerebral cortex determined by Krypton 85. *Acta physiol. Scand.* 54, 325 (1962).
26. Heiss, W. D., Gerstenbrand, F., Prosenz, P. & Krenn, J., The prognostic value of cerebral blood flow measurement in patients with the apallic syndrome. *J. neurol. Sci.* 16, 373 (1972).
27. McDowall, D. G., The effects of clinical concentrations of halothane on the blood flow and oxygen uptake of the cerebral cortex. *Brit. J. Anaesth.* 39, 186 (1967).
28. Wollman, H., Alexander, S. C., Cohen, P. J., Smith, T. C., Chase, P. E. & van der

Molen R. A., Cerebral circulation during general anesthesia and hyperventilation in man. *Anaesthesiology* 26, 329 (1965).

29. Nilsson, E. & Ingvar, D. H., Cerebral blood flow during neurolept-analgesia in the cat. *Acta. anaesth. Scand.* 10, 47 (1966).

30. Freeman, J. & Ingvar, D. H., Effect of Fentanyl on cerebral cortical blood flow and EEG in the cat. *Acta. anaesth. Scand.* 11, 381 (1967).

31. Kucher, R., Benzer, H., Böck, F., Brenner, H., Eisterer, H., Gerstenbrand, F., Haider, W., Klenn, J., Lackner, F., Mostbeck, A., Niessner, G., Pateisky, K., Prosenz, P., Riede, W., Schultes, L., Sigmar, L., Steinbereithner, K., Tschakaloff, C., Zeitelberger, P. & Valenczak, E., *Zur Längsschnittbeurteilung schwerer Schädel-Hirnverletzter.* Proc. 4. Fortb. kurs klin. Anaesth., Wien 1969.

32. Holzman, G. B., Wagner, H. N., Ilo, M., Rabonowitz, D. & Zierler, K. L., Measurement of muscle blood flow in the human forearm with radioactive krypton and xenon. *Circulation* 30, 27 (1964).

33. Kloster, F. E., Bristow, J. D. & Griswold, H. E., Cardiac output determination from precordial isotope-dilution curves during exercise. *J. appl. Physiol.* 26, 465 (1969).

34. Bergman, S., Siegel, I. A. & Ciancio, S., Absorption of Carbon-14-labeled Lidocaine through the oral mucosa. *J. D. Res.* 47, 1184 (1968).

35. van Dyke R. A., Chenoweth, M. B. & Larsen, E. R., Synthesis and metabolism of Halothane-1-C^{14}. *Nature,* 204, 471 (1964).

36. Höfer, R., Krenn, J. Pfeiffer, G. & Steinbereithner, K., Untersuchungen zur Ausscheidung von Diallyl-nor-Toxiferin bei Nierentransplantation, *Anaesthesist,* 18, 304 (1969).

37. Cohen, E. N., Brewer, H. W. & Smith, D., The metabolism and elimination of d-tubocurarine-^{3}H. *Anesthesiology* 28, 309 (1967).

38. Dal Santo, G., Kinetics of distribution of radioactive labelled muscle relaxants, I. Investigation with ^{14}C-dimethyl-d-tubocurarine. *Anesthesiology* 25, 788 (1964).

39. Krenn, J. & Steinbereithner, K., *Anaesthesieprobleme bei der Nierentransplantation.* Proc. 4. Fortbildungskurs klin. Anaesth., Wien 1969.

40. Chinard, F. P. & Enns, T., Transcapillary pulmonary exchange of water in the dog. *Amer. J. Physiol.* 178, 197 (1954).

41. Lowenstein, E., Travis, K., Malt, R. A. & Laver, M. B., Substitution of iodoantipyrine-I^{131} (IAP) for H^3O in the pulmonary extravascular water (PEVW) measurement. *Fed. Proc.* 28, 281 (1969).

42. Gump, F. E., Mashima, Y. & Kinney, J. M., Water balance and extravascular lung water measurements in surgical patients. *Amer. J. Surg.* 119, 515 (1970).

43. Pontoppidan, H., Geffin, B. & Lowenstein, E., Acute respiratory failure in the adult. (I) *N. Engl. J. Med.* 287, 690 (1972).

44. Ebaugh, F. G., Emerson, C. P. & Ross, J. F., The use of radioactive chromium 51 as an erythrocyte tagging agent for the determination of red cell survival in vivo. *J. clin Invest.* 32, 1260 (1953).

45. Kühböck, J., Lauringer, P., Zeitelberger, P. & Zekert, F., Untersuchungen zur Genese der Anämie von Schädelhirnverletzten. *Anaesthesist* 20, 398, (1971).

46. Kronenberg, R. S., L'Heureux, P., Ponto, R. A., Drage, C. W. & Loken, M. K., The effect of aging on lung perfusion. *Ann. int. Med.* 76, 413 (1972).

47. Ingrisch, H., Heinze, H. G., Pfeifer, K. J. & Lissner, J., Lungenfunktions-Szintigraphie mit ^{133}Xenon. *Münch. med. Wschr.* 115, 341 (1973).

48. Rösler, H., Ramos, M., Kinser, J., Hoffmann, W., Schnaars, P. & Zuppinger, A., Die ^{133}Xe/^{99m}Tc-MAP-Lungenszintigraphie. *Schweiz. med. Wschr.* 103, 857 (1973).

49. Strieder, D. J., Barnes, B. A., Aronow, S., Russell, P. S. & Kazemi, H., Xenon 133 study of ventilation and perfusion in transplanted dog lungs. *J. appl. Physiol.* 23, 359 (1967).

50. West, J. B. & Dollery, C. T., Absorption of inhaled radioactive water vapor. *Nature* 189, 588 (1961).
51. Wolfsdorf, J. & Swift, D., Isotope scanning in the comparison of the deposition of radioactive aqueous aerosols delivered by jet or ultrasonic nebulizers to the respiratory tract. Abstracts Soc. Ped. Res., May 1968, quoted from Graff, D. T., Benson, D. W.: Systemic and pulmonary changes with inhaled humid atmospheres. *Anesthesiology* 30, 199 (1969).

MEASUREMENT OF NEUROMUSCULAR BLOCK

S. A. FELDMAN

Although it is possible to measure the degree of impairment of neuro-muscular transmission in animals and man, unfortunately it is impossible to obtain a direct quantitative measure of the activity of muscle relaxants at this site. Indeed the simplicity with which it is possible to measure the muscular weakness induced by muscle relaxants makes it only too easy to conclude that this represents a quantitative picture of the activity of these drugs; this assumption has led to misleading and erroneous deductions.

The early appreciation of the marked species difference in sensitivity to the muscle relaxant drugs made us aware that it is not relevant to extrapolate from measurements of muscle paralysis induced in animals to what might occur in man. Zaimis (1) drew attention to the differences that occurred in the response of animals to decamethonium. Generally animals that are more sensitive to depolarising muscle relaxants than man, exhibit resistance to non-depolarising drugs and vice versa. Zaimis was of the opinion that of all the small experimental animals, the cat most closely resembled man in its sensitivity to depolarising and non-depolarising drugs. Today it is usual to test muscle relaxants of Rhesus monkeys as it has been found that, although the quantitative sensitivity of the cat to depolarising and non-depolarising drugs is similar to man, the duration of a drugs activity can be better assessed in this animal than in the cat.

Not only is it impossible to extrapolate from the results obtained in animals species to man, but it is probable that there is considerable variation between seemingly otherwise similar experimental animals and between patients (2, 3) (Fig. 1). It is probable that differences also occur between different groups of muscles in the same individual, and even possibly in the same muscle group in the same individual from day to day.

With these reservations in mind, it is obvious that the potential sources of error and misunderstanding are great. Indeed it is difficult to obtain truly reproducible conditions and biological error is unavoidable. To minimise this error wherever possible, measurements of neuromuscular block should

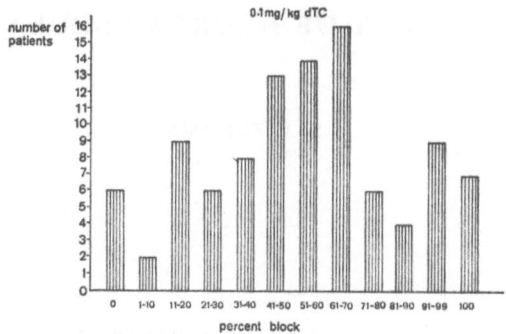

Fig. 1. Effect of 0,1 mg/kg of tubocurarine on twitch hight in 100 patients. (Note marked variation in percentage block produced by this dose). From Katz (3).

be made on the same muscle group in the same patient or animal on the same day.

Once one has obtained a measurement of muscle response to indirect stimulation it is tempting to assume that any reduction of this response consequent upon administration of a muscle relaxant drug is quantitatively proportional to the action of that drug at the drug-receptor site. This is unfortunately not so.

Blockage of neuromuscular transmission by muscle relaxant drugs cannot be demonstrated unless there is over 50 % receptor occupancy. Thus it is impossible to measure the quantitative effect of small doses of relaxant drug. Paton and Waud (4) showed that it was not possible to detect a diminution in twitch response following supramaximal stimulation of a motor nerve, unless over 70 % of the receptors were occupied by curare. Complete neuromuscular block occurred at 90 % receptor occupancy (Fig. 2). As a result, if one is using faradic stimulation no effect will be seen until three quarters of the receptors have been occluded by drug; minor degrees of drug-receptor reaction cannot therefore be detected by this means.

In later experiments (5) it was demonstrated that, if tetanic rates of motor nerve stimulation were used, lesser degrees of receptor occupancy could be detected but even using grossly unphysiological stimulation rates of 200 Hz, it was impossible to reveal less than 50 % receptor occupancy (Fig. 3).

It is obviously impossible to measure the subclinical activity of the muscle relaxants by measuring the effect on muscle contraction. Indeed, when one watches an indirectly evoked muscle twitch recover from 100 % paralysis to complete recovery one is only seeing the tip of an iceberg emerge, the bulk of the effect remains unmeasured.

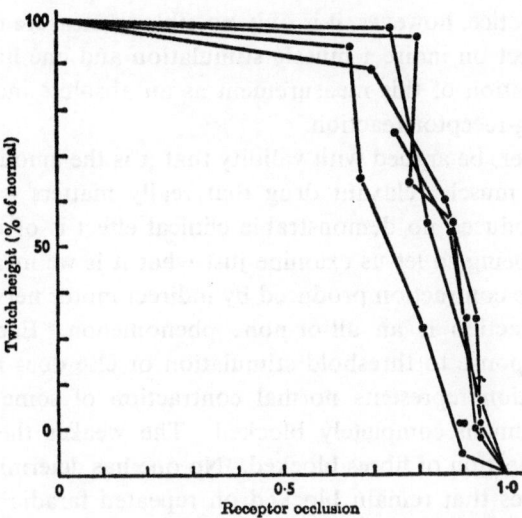

Fig. 2. Receptor occlusion required to suppress twitch response. From Paton & Waud (4).

In experiments which I have performed using gallamine one can demonstrate this residual undetected receptor occlusion, 2 hours after apparent complete recovery of twitch height, by noticing the positive additive effect of a second dose of a non-depolarising relaxant, a cumulative phenomenon.

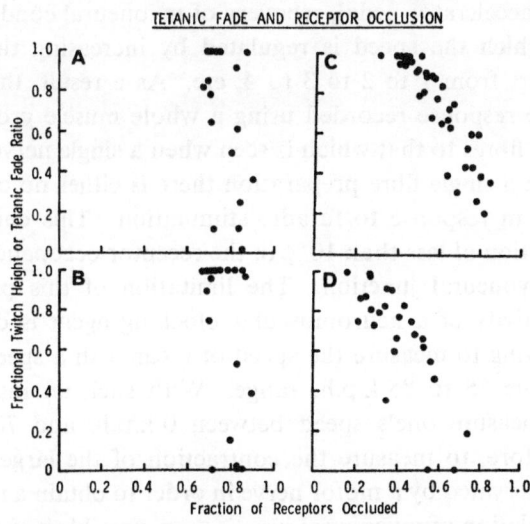

Fig. 3. Relation between twitch response (A), tetanic fade (B, C and D) and receptor occlusion. Tetanic stimulation 30 (B), 100 (C) and 200 Hz (D). From Waud & Waud (5).

In clinical practice, however, it is only possible to measure neuromuscular block by its effect on indirect muscle stimulation and one has therefore to accept the limitation of this measurement as an absolute indication of the quantity of drug-receptor reaction.

It can, however, be argued with validity that it is the amount of paralysis produced by a muscle relaxant drug that really matters – drug-receptor activity that produced no demonstrable clinical effect is of no clinical importance. This being so let us examine just what it is we measure when we study the muscle contraction produced by indirect motor nerve stimulation.

Muscle contraction is an all-or-none phenomenon. Each fibre either contracts in response to threshold stimulation or else does not. A partial muscle contraction represents normal contraction of some muscle fibres whilst others remain completely blocked. The weaker the response the greater the proportion of fibres blocked. No one has determined whether it is the same fibres that remain blocked on repeated faradic stimulation or whether there is a rotation of contracting fibres. The muscle fade that occurs on tetanic stimulation after exposure to a non-depolarising relaxant suggests that some fibres 'tire' easily, needing a greater release of acetylcholine to trigger off their contraction.

Recovery of twitch response following myoneural block therefore represents a slow increase in the number of fibres responding to the acetylcholine discharge from the motor nerve. Unlike a motor car whose speed varies with pressure on the accelerator pedal, recovery of myoneural conduction resembles a car in which the speed is regulated by increasing the number of working cylinders from 1 to 2 to 3 to 4, etc. As a result, there is a basic difference in the response recorded using a whole muscle group or even a group of muscle fibres to that which is seen when a single nerve muscle fibre is studied. With a single fibre preparation there is either no contraction or full contraction in response to faradic stimulation. This change possibly reflects a diminution of less than 10% in the receptor occupancy by relaxant drug at that myoneural junction. The limitation of this preparation in assessing the activity of a neuromuscular blocking agent is obvious. It is equivalent to trying to measure the speed of a car with a speedometer that only recorded the 75 to 85 k.p.h. range. With such an instrument it is impossible to measure one's speed between 0 k.p.h. and 70 k.p.h. It is preferable therefore, to measure the contraction of the largest number of muscle fibres innervated by a motor nerve in order to obtain a response from as varied a population of myoneural junctions as possible and thus to widen the range of receptor activity that may affect muscle contraction.

MEASURING MUSCLE CONTRACTIONS

Most of the work recording the effect of muscle contraction in patients and volunteers has been the result of studies using apparatus that allow free shortening of the muscle to occur – isotonic contraction. This is the normal purpose of most muscle groups, other than those concerned with posture. The disadvantage of measuring isotonic contraction is that the resultant twitch will depend upon the mechanical efficiency of the muscle group studied and the results cannot therefore be extrapolated, in a quantitatively meaningful sense, to other muscles. There is also unlikely to be a linear relationship between the height of the twitch produced and the effectiveness of neuromuscular conduction, just as it would not be expected for there to be a direct linear relationship between the number of men pushing a car and the speed produced. It is only over a relatively narrow section of the response that any degree of linearity might be anticipated, that is, once the car had started to move and before it approached the maximum speed. It is usual therefore when using isotonic or semi-isotonic recording systems to measure the slope of the middle half of the recovery, i.e. the 25 to 75 % recovery time (Fig. 4).

Isometric contraction offers a better index for the measurement of the number of muscle fibres contracting in response to a motor nerve stimulation. Provided one uses it to study the effect of neuromuscular block upon a muscle that is physiological postural in nature. The strain gauge caliper used by Zaimis, Cannard and Price (6) (Fig. 5) in their studies on the effect of temperature on muscle relaxants, is basically isometric and therefore should give better quantitative results. Unfortunately my own efforts with this apparatus, stimulating the anterior tibial nerve, evoked both direct and indirect muscle response and made it difficult to interpret the resulting increase in tension in the muscle.

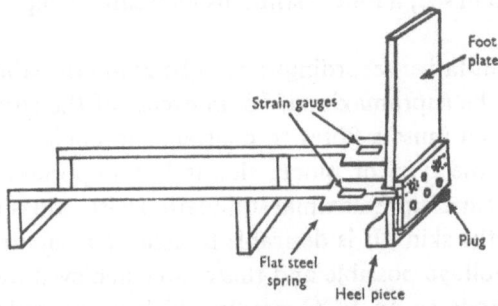

Fig. 5. Strain gauge caliper used by Zaimis et al. (6) to study isometric contraction of tibialis anterior in humans. From Churchill Davidson, H. C. & Wylie, D. A., Practice of anaesthesia (Lloyd Luke).

In animal experiments it is far simpler to achieve a truly isometric preparation and to measure the resulting increase in tension resulting from indirect stimulation.

The use of the stretched diaphragm preparation, stimulated through the phrenic nerve, has also given results that are difficult to interpret. Although the preparation is isometric, the muscle was never intended to function in this fashion and the tension generated is believed to cause early deterioration in the preparation. It should be pointed out that this common pharmacological preparation differs from any in vivo situation for three reasons:

1. it is not perfused through arteries, any drug has to reach the site of action by diffusion from the water bath into the muscle,
2. its oxygenation depends upon diffusion from the surface and is probably insufficient, in the thick rat diaphragm, which is passively exercised by repeated tetanic stimulation,
3. drug introduced into the water bath remains at a constant concentration. In the in vivo preparation the blood level would fall due to redistribution, excretion and metabolism.

This preparation is suited principally for short experiments, for example, to demonstrate reversal of action of relaxant; it is less suited for recovery measurements as it cannot be regarded as a true model of an 'in vivo' situation.

STIMULATION ARTEFACTS

Motor nerve stimulation requires threshold depolarisation of its surface. This requires a voltage of 5-10 V directly applied to the nerve. The duration of the stimulus should be as brief as possible to produce the required ionic flux, i.e. 0.2 to 0.5 m sec; a longer stimulus may cause a biphasic or repetitive stimulus.

Whenever quantitative recordings are to be made the stimulus applied to the nerve should be supramaximal, i.e. in excess of the current required to cause all innervated muscle fibres to contract. In clinical practice, such as the diagnosis of the type of block, this is less important. It may prove impossible to obtain a supramaximal stimulation with skin surface electrodes, without burning the skin. It is desirable to achieve a supramaximal current with the lowest voltage possible and this can be achieved by connecting the stimulating electrode to an ECG needle which is inserted subcutaneously parallel to the nerve. This avoids the large and variable skin resistance element. The needle should not be inserted with its point towards the nerve to prevent the high charge density at the tip from burning the nerve.

For accurate quantitative comparisons it is essential to ensure that, when a single stimulus is applied to a nerve, a single maximal discharge of acetylcholine is produced. In the case of most peripheral nerves this necessitates preventing secondary effects due to reflex stimulation causing repetitive firing, by either crushing or cutting the nerve proximal to the point of stimulation or alternatively applying a local anaesthetic block proximal to the point of stimulation.

This does not mean to imply that perfectly valid conclusions about the presence or absence of drug activity cannot be obtained using a stimulator that delivers a wide pulse of a lower voltage when afferent nerve impulses have not been blocked – provided that comparisons are only made on the same preparation, with the same apparatus at that time. The limitation of the use of non-supramaximal stimuli is to know how many fibres are discharging. If all the nerve fibres are stimulated by a supramaximal stimulus, this can easily be reproduced on another occasion. If an unkown proportion only are stimulated, this cannot be reproduced quantitatively at a later date.

MEASURING DEVICES

The isometric apparatus used in animal experiments is unsuitable for man. The most successful apparatus that has been used in man is the foot caliper of Zaimis et al. (6).

Isotonic apparatus – commonest and most convenient to use

A. *Ergometrics* – depending upon voluntary power of a volunteer to squeeze a bulb connected to a column of mercury or a pressure transducer. This simple apparatus requires careful fixation of the hand as the extensors of the wrist are less readily paralysed than the flexor muscles.

The use of tidal volume measurements to indicate the degree of diaphragmatic paralysis has given useful clinical results. It is simple to use but limited in its application as the tidal volume is affected not only by muscle weakness but also by respiratory centre drive. Thus, depression of the respiratory centre by general anaesthesia will give a resulting diminution in tidal volume identical to that produced by a muscle relaxant. Conversely diminution in tidal volume produced by a muscle relaxant will cause CO_2 accumulation and increased respiratory drive antagonising the depression of tidal volume produced by a muscle relaxant, as the usual phrenic nerve activity is less than supramaximal.

B. *Force displacement transducers* for measurement of contraction of adductor pollicis longus and brevis muscles (Fig. 6). This apparatus is simple to use, the one illustrated can be applied to a thumb in a few minutes. This apparatus described by Tyrrell (7) uses a Statham UC3 load cell and has proved to be reliable and effective.

ELECTROMYOGRAPHY

This technique records the compound action potential from a group of contracting muscles and is displayed upon an oscilloscope. On superficial theoretical consideration it has been suggested that this should parallel the muscle contraction produced. Katz (8) pointed out that, somewhat surprisingly, the results of studies using electromyography may differ from those obtained using a strain gauge to measure indirect stimulation of the same muscle, under certain circumstances.

Measurements of neuromuscular conduction are relatively simple to make. However, the information obtained has to be very carefully interpreted before speculating about the effect of muscle relaxant drugs, in view of the limitations of the apparatus used and the pharmacological and physiological basis of the effect to be measured. It must be remembered that:

a. it does not necessarily reflect the drug-receptor reaction in a quantitative manner;
b. it depends upon the method of stimulation, the muscle stimulated and the type of muscle activity recorded;
c. it varies according to whether electrical or mechanical recording method is used;
d. it does not necessarily reflect the response of all muscles in that individual, nor in the same muscle in different individuals or species.

REFERENCES

1. Zaimis, E. J., Motor and plate differences as a determining factor in the mode of action of neuromuscular blocking substances. *Nature (London)* 170, 617 (1952).
2. Nastuck, W. L. & Alving, B.O., Further studies of edrophonium and its close analogues with respect to activity at neuromuscular junction. *Biochem. Pharmacol.* 1, 307 (1958).
3. Katz, R. L., Monitoring of muscle relaxation and neuromuscular transmission. In: *Patient monitoring* edited by Crul, J. F. & Payne, J. P. Exerpta Medica, Amsterdam 1970.
4. Paton, W. D. M. & Waud, D. R., Margin of safety of muscle relaxant drugs. *J. Physiol. Lond.* 191, 59 (1947).

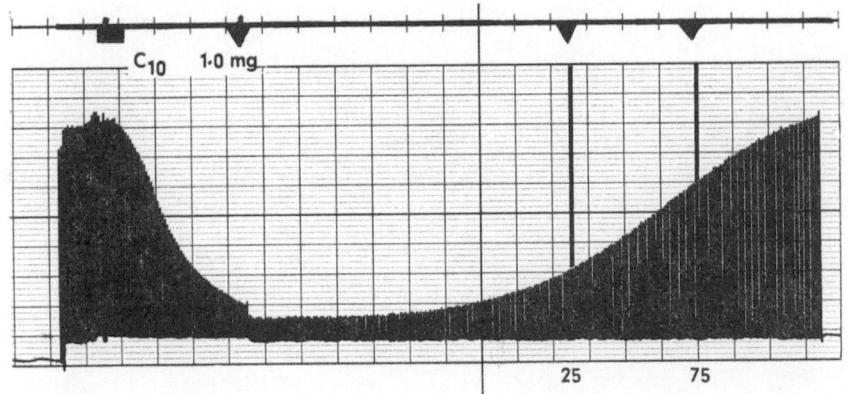

Fig. 4. Recovery slope following decamethonium. Isotonic recording. Note lack of linearity of recovery slope. The use of 25% to 75% recovery time introduces an index of recovery for quantatative comparison.

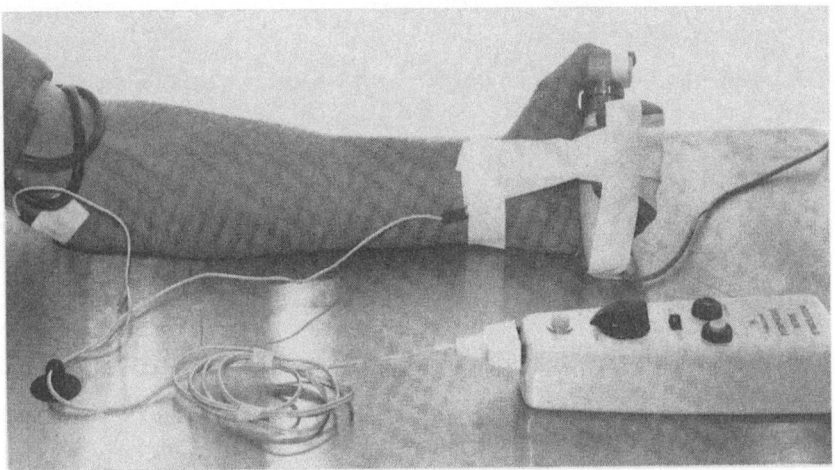

Fig. 6. A simple apparatus for the measurement of the force of thumb adduction using a Statham UC3 force displacement transducer mounted in a bicycle handle grip – after Tyrrell (7).

5. Waud, B. E. & Waud, D. R., The relation between tetanic fade and receptor occlusion in the presence of competitive neuromuscular block. *Anaesthesiology* 35, 456 (1971).
6. Zaimis, E. J., Cannard, T. H. & Price. H. L., Effects of lowered muscle temperature on neuromuscular blockade in man. *Science* 128, 34 (1958).
7. Tyrrell, M. F. The measurement of the force of thumb adduction. *Anaesthesia* 24, 626 (1969).
8. Katz, R. L., *Neuromuscular pharmacology of suxamethonium*. Report to Faculty of Anaesthetists, Royal College of Surgeons – Study Day, 1973.

THE MEASUREMENT OF PAIN:

THE ANAESTHETIST

JOH. SPIERDIJK, W. T. C. D. CORNET AND W. J. KWEEKEL–DE VRIES

The anaesthetist uses pain-relieving drugs not only during anaesthesia but also for premedication, during the postoperative period and for his work in the pain clinic. When choosing his drugs, the anaesthetist will turn to the pharmacologist who can compare the action of various drugs in animal experiments and to the clinical pharmacologist who extends these tests to man.

We all know that psychological components play a role in pain. This is true in the pain clinic and also before, during and after surgery. Eikenbroek in our department has investigated the relationship between preoperative fear and postoperative pain. If we understand clinical pain to mean 'the reaction of the whole personality to the pain-producing lesion', then the complexity inherent in the measurement of pain immediately becomes clear. Pain is a sensation. Each sensation has a local, temporal, quantitative and qualitative aspect. These sensation parameters of one single sensory experience are in fact much more complex because they are normally experienced as a combination of many simultaneous sensations which are compared not only with one another but also with those previously experienced as well as those anticipated in the future (1). The concept that pain is composed of cognitive as well as affective components has led to attempts to measure the original sensation and the reaction to pain as two separate phenomena (2). In spite of intensive research, physical objective standards to indicate the degree of pain have not yet been found (3). Most investigators (4) are critical of 'measurements' of pain. The purpose of these measurements is to express in numbers the degree to which a certain intensity of pain differs from a set norm or basic value. This is, in their opinion, not feasible since before quantitative concepts can be considered, it must first be possible to define precisely such changes as worse – same – less severe; although it would seem that this is a simple matter, it appears in practice that numerous problems are ncountered, Moreover, it has also been shown that as far as pain stimuli are concerned, the same stimulus in different areas or in the same area under various conditions gives different responses. If, therefore even the (objective) assessment of pain in the sense of worse – same – less, is difficult, then according to many authors changes in pain can also not be expressed quantitatively.

One should therefore be critical of measurements of sensibility or pain as well as quantitative terms to express feelings which develop as a result of the stimulation of certain receptors. Just as hunger and thirst cannot be recorded in numbers, except possibly in terms of what is required to satiate these states, neither can pain be expressed in numbers.

The symptoms which accompany pain can be grouped as follows:

a. spinal reflexes in acute pain (e.g. withdrawal of the hand from thermal stimuli);
b. autonomic reflexes: these signs in particular help the anaesthetist determine pain during anaesthesia when these symptoms may also be present;
   1. tachycardia
   2. increase in blood pressure
   3. lacrimation – perspiration
   4. hyperpnea
c. psychological reaction of patients to pain (e.g. fear, depression, agression, distress and frustration).

However, a quantitative relationship between any one of these symptoms and the degree of pain has never been demonstrated. The degree of pain is dependent upon central physiological factors such as inhibition and facilitation and psychogenic factors such as personality, experience and memory, as well as external conditions.

Most investigators limit themselves to measurement of the decrease in pain. For these measurements, they reason that a verbal report of the patient is the most reliable and simplest index of pain. In general therefore the investigator is also dependent upon the willingness of the patient to communicate. Observations based on non-verbal reactions of the patient (facial expression, perspiration, tachycardia etc.) are considered without value. It appears that in general graded quantification is preferred for measurement of pain instead of the so-called 'yes or no' approach (5). The latter method, which in short means that groups of patients are studied to determine the percentage with total pain relief after administration of analgesics in varying dosages, seems to be simple but in practice many insurmountable objections are encountered. For 'graded measurement', the approach is as follows: the patient is requested to categorize his pain as light, moderate or unbearable. This is repeated after administration of the analgesic or placebo at set intervals (6). In this case, the simplest scoring system is to consider each progression from one level to the next as a unit. This can easily be recorded graphically.

In the foregoing methods, most measurements rely on the subjective response of the patient and are obtained by verbal response or use of a signal box (with the same result) (1). In addition another approach, involving the use of more objective data, has become fashionable.

Analgesics administered postoperatively can cause an improvement in ventilation (by decreasing pain) but also depression of breathing (central). Still, by using long function tests and determination of blood gas values, it is possible to compare the effectiveness of various analgesics (7, 8, 9). In its purest form, this comparison can be made while using local techniques to relieve pain because there is no depression of the respiratory center (10, 11). Alexander, Parik and Spence of Glasgow (12) compared the effect after upper abdominal surgery of the administration of

A. 45 mg pentazocine i.m. on demand;

B. 45 mg pentazocine i.m. every 4 hours for 48 hours;

C. 540 mg pentazocine via continuous intravenous infusion for 48 hours;

D. 10 mg morphine i.m. on demand;

E. 10 mg morphine i.m. every 4 hours for 48 hours.

Functional residual capacity and vital capacity, alveolar and arterial oxygen tension and PCO_2 were measured.

They found that there is a greater difference in alveolar/arterial oxygen tension during the first 5 days after upper abdominal surgery. The PCO_2 is elevated during the first 2 postoperative days while PO_2 is decreased.

It was found that patients who were given analgesics by regular injection or infusion received considerably more drugs than those on other regimens However, there was only a marginal improvement in the pulmonary gas exchange in comparison with those on more conventional medication.

To date, these authors are under the impression that clinically the patiesnt on a regular regimen are more comfortable.

The Glasgow group concluded that it is possible to compare different kinds of drug regimens using the lung function tests.

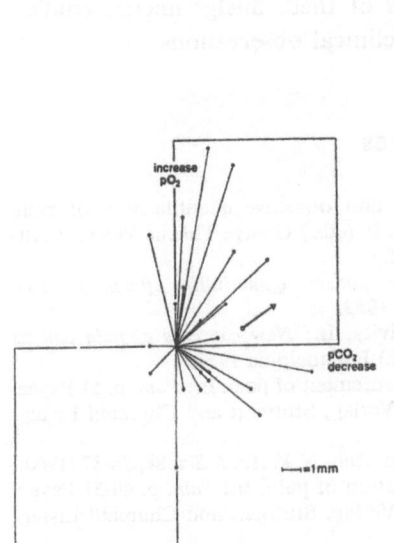

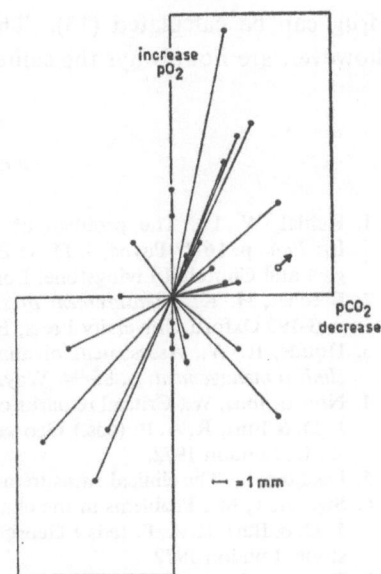

Fig. 1. The influence on PO$_2$ and PCO$_2$ after an injection of 2 mg lysine acetylsalicylate.

Fig. 2. The influence on PO$_2$ and PCO$_2$ after an injection of 10 mg of morphine.

In 51 gynaecological patients, we compared the effect on postoperative pain of an injectable salicylate (1,8 g lysine acetylsalicylate – equivalent to 1 g acetylsalicylic acid and 10 mg morphine, both administered intramuscularly (13, 14). We observed no difference in activity, measured as pain intensity and subjective pain relief scores. It even appeared that 1,8 g lysine acetylsalicylate works faster than 10 mg morphine. We also found that detrimental side-effects such as vomiting and nausea are less frequent with lysine acetylsalicylate. The effect on blood gas values is, however, much more difficult to interpret. In this case, various effects merge together, namely the pain decreases and therefore the patient breathes easier. Aspirin stimulates the respiratory center whereas morphine inhibits it.

The drop in PCO$_2$ is greater after administration of lysine acetylsalicylate than after a morphine injection (Fig 1)

Besides there is an increase in PO$_2$ observed after administration of morphine as well as after lysine acetylsalicylate (Fig. 2).

In conclusion: precise analgesimetry during anaesthesia as well as the postoperative period is not possible. With the help of postoperative lung function tests it is possible to compare different drug regimens. Furthermore the therapeutic equivalence of different routes of administration of the same drug can be calculated (15). The results of these analgesimetric studies, however, are not always the same as our clinical observations

REFERENCES

1. Keidel, W. D., The problem of subjective and objective quantification of pain. In: *Pain.* p. 16-27 Payne, J. D. & Burt, R. A. P. (eds.) George Thieme Verlag, Stuttgart and Churchill Livingstone, London 1972.
2. Beecher, H. K., *Measurement of subjective responses: Quantitative effects of drugs.* p. 3-190 Oxford University Press, New York 1959.
3. Houde, R. W., Assessment of analgetic activity. In: *New concepts of pain and its clinical management.* p. 85-94. Way, E. L. (ed.) Philadelphia 1967.
4. Noordenbos, W., Critical remarks on the measurement of pain. In: *Pain.* p. 51 Payne, J. D. & Burt, R. A. P. (eds.) George Thieme Verlag, Stuttgart and Churchill Livingstone, London 1972.
5. Lasagna, L., The clinical measurement of pain. *Ann. N.Y. Acad. Sci.* 86, 28-37 (1960).
6. Swerdlow, M., Problems in the clinical evaluation of pain. In: *Pain.* p. 49-51 Payne, J. D. & Burt, R. A. P. (eds.) George Thieme Verlag, Stuttgart and Churchill Livingstone, London 1972.
7. Diamant, M. L. & Palmer, K., Postoperative changes in the gas tensions of arterial blood and ventilatory function. *Lancet* 23, 180 (1966).
8. Bromage, P. R., Spirometry in assessment of analgesia after abdominal surgery. *Brit. Med. J.* vol. II, 589 (1955).
9. Mayrhofer, K., Blutgasanalytische Vergleichsuntersuchungen bei Verwendung von Analgetika zur Bekämpfung des postoperativen Wundschmerze. In: *Proceedings 1st Europ. Congress of Anaesthesiology* I, chapter 22, Wien 1962.
10. Bergman, H. & Necek, St., Respiratorische Vergleichsuntersuchungen bei epiduraler und zentraler postoperativer Analgesie. In: *Postoperative Schmerzbekämpfung.* Ber. V. Int. Bremer NLA-Symp. 1971 I p. 27-39 Henschel, W. F. (Hrsg.) Stuttgart 1972.
11. Wurster, J. & Nolte, H., Postoperative Analgesie und Lungenfunktion. In: *Postoperative Schmerzbekämpfung.* Ber. V. Int. Bremer NLA-Symp. 1971 I p. 43-48 Henschel, W. F. (Hrsg.) Stuttgart 1972.
12. Alexander, J. L. Parikh, R. K., Spence, A. A., Postoperative analgesia and lungfunction: a comparison of narcotic analgesia regimens. *Brit. J. Anaesth.* 43, 346 (1973).
13. Lelkens, J. P. M. & Geigeratt, R. A., A comparison of the effects of intramuscular and rectal administration of pentazocine isung pH and pCO_2 measurements. In: *Proceedings, Vth world congress of anaesthesiologists,* Kyoto 1972, Excerpta Medica, Amsterdam 1974.
14. Spierdijk, J. & Kweekel–de Vries, W. J., Experiences with Bezitramide (an oral morphinomimetic) and Aspegic (a parenteral acetylsalicylate). Multidisciplinary approach to pain patients in Leiden University Hospital. In: *Proceedings, Vth world congress of anaesthesiologists,* Kyoto 1972, p. 270. Excerpta Medica, Amsterdam 1974.
15. Kweekel–de Vries, W. J., Hermans, J. M. H., Mattie, H. & Spierdijk, J., A new soluble acetylsalicylic acid derivative in the treatment of postoperative pain (to be published).

THE MEASUREMENT OF PAIN:

THE PSYCHOLOGIST

H. J. EIKENBROEK

When we talk about measuring pain, what we have in mind is a sort of ideal instrument or else a physiological indicator which would enable us to objectively define the intensity of pain. A satisfactory physiological indicator of pain would be one which is present (or increased) when pain is felt, and absent (or reduced) when pain is not felt. As it is, there is at present no single accepted indicator of pain that can be counted to vary in an orderly way with degrees of pain and absence of pain. A seemingly objective measure may have to be contrasted with the patient's subjective statement about his pain perception and, much to our regret, we have to note that up to date the only reliable, sound measure of pain we have at our disposal, is the information which the patient himself gives about his perception of pain.

If, however, we want to put our trust in the use of the physiological indicator without the supportive verbal reports of the patient, then we shall find that when testing the validity of such an indicator – and why should we otherwise take the trouble to find an indicator at all – we cannot forego the verbal statements made by the patient about the pain he feels. In other words: we shall have to establish the correlation between the physiological indicator and the patient's verbal report.

How far can we trust the patient when he tells us about the amount of pain he experiences? In order to establish the reliability of the patient's expression of his pain we must go into the laboratory and in this setting the subjective statements can be tested against the experimentally produced pain stimuli. One method by which we can do this is by applying a highly controllable electrocutaneous stimulation technique. The electrical and physical properties of this system have been stabilised by use of a controlled current stimulator and a concentric shock electrode. This shock electrode consists of a plastic casing with an inner aluminum disc surrounded by a concentric aluminum annulus. The concentric electrode form circumscribes the surface area through which current flows, thus ensuring a more constant area of tissue stimulation than is obtained with other arrangements. An added advantage of this electrode is that it reduces the extraneous sensations produced by tetany. These factors, in conjunction with a method for stabilizing skin impedance under the electrode at 5000 ohms, ensures the electrical and physical stability of the system.

Tursky and O'Connell (1) have investigated the reliability of subjective judgements by laboratory experiments in which three concentric shock electrodes were placed on the dorsal surface of the subject's forearm. The 10 volunteer subjects for this experiment were asked to make judgements about four qualitatively defined levels of intensity. The designations of the four levels and the instructions used were as follows:

1. *Threshold Level.* We are going to present a series of stimuli of increasing intensity. Tell us when you feel any sensation under the electrode on your right (or left) arm.
2. *Discomfort Level.* We shall gradually increase the intensity of the stimulation until you consider the sensation to be uncomfortable.
3. *Painful Level.* Now we will gradually increase the intensity of the stimulus until you consider the sensation to be painful.
4. *Tolerance Level.* Now we will gradually increase the intensity of the stimulation until you tell us that you don't want to go any higher.

Runs were begun with an initial intensity of 0,1 mA, below threshold for all subjects. Shocks were of 1 sec duration and spaced about 20 sec apart. The intensity was then raised to the closest higher multiple of 0,5 mA and increased on each successive shock by steps of 0,5 mA until tolerance level was reached. A simple run consisted of determinations of all four levels on all electrodes by this procedure. Five successive runs were made on each of 2 days scheduled at least a week apart. The basic measures were the shock intensities in milliamperes at each of the four judgement levels and for the average of the three electrodes. The first set of correlations computed consisted of comparisons from run to run within each day. All 60 within-day correlations for the uncomfortable, painful and tolerance levels ranged from 0,85 to 1,00 and were all significant at a 0,001 level of significance. Six of the 20 correlations for the threshold level were not significant, indicating lower reliability at this level of intensity. The second set of correlations was made between runs on the two successive days. For each judgement level, each run on the first day was correlated with each of the five runs on the second day, thus yielding 25 correlations for each judgement level. Of the 75 day to day correlations for the uncomfortable, painful and tolerance levels, 59 correlations were significant at an 0,005 level and the remaining 16 at p < ,01. However, 23 of the 25 correlations for the threshold level were not statistically significant.

These findings strongly suggest that it is in any case possible to give reliable subjective statements of nociceptive sensations in a laboratory setting. Can studies conducted in the laboratory contribute to the needs of the clinician outside the walls of the laboratory? Beecher (2) argues that experimental pain is not identical to pathological pain. He warns against simply generalising findings from the experimental situation to the clinical situation. It has been demonstrated that the severity of the pain following a surgical operation is not only influenced by the wound itself but also by the patient's reaction to this wound. As regards the pain experienced the significance of the wound is of great importance and therefore pain in an experimental situation has a different meaning to the subject than pain perceived by the patient in a clinical situation.

There is, however, no reason to assume, that the patient's subjective report of his pain should in any way be less reliable than the evaluation of pain given by the experimental subject.

There is a great variation in the amount of pain reported by different individuals who have undergone similar surgical operations and their reportings must be regarded as reliable. But also experimental subjects show considerable individual differences as regards their perception of pain and will express it by using terms such as uncomfortable, painful, intolerable even though the shock intensities administered were the same for all subjects. The aforementioned experiments have revealed that whereas one subject will experience a shock intensity of 6 mA as uncomfortable, another subject, given the same intensity of shock, will report an unbearable pain experience. Both evaluations relating to pain should, however, be considered as highly reliable. Thus, the sensation of pain as we know it through the patient's verbal reports, will not only be determined by nociceptive stimulation, but also by a great number of other factors to which Beecher (2) assigns the term 'reaction component'. Consequently, the painscore will reflect a sensation component as well as a reaction component. It is this reaction component which suggests that, among other things, anxiety is a significant factor in the experience of pain.

Another study dealing with the problem of pain was designed to assess the relationship between neuroticism scores, that is scores measuring emotional stability and proneness to anxiety, and pain. Findings of this study indicate that in general, patients with a low neuroticism score, that is, people who are emotionally stable and not unduly prone to anxiety, will experience less pain than those with a high N-score.

Recent investigations by Parbrook et al. (3) demonstrated that patients with a low N-score have less postoperative pain than patients with a high N-score. To quote: '...there is little doubt that anxious patients are likely to have more severe pain'.

Here in Leiden Eikenbroek and Herzberg (4) have attempted to measure anxiety by a more direct method to assess how far preoperative anxiety bears a relationship on postoperative pain. The subjects chosen for this experiment were 45 female patients who underwent comparable gynaecological operations. The patients were seen the night before scheduled surgery and given the Amsterdam version of the Wolpe and Lang Fear Survey Schedule. This fear inventory comprises 128 items, including such items as 'being alone,' 'witnessing a surgical operation' 'thunderstorms', 'hospital smells', 'being alone in an elevator', 'germs' and 'dead people'. All these items refer to situations, things, people that may cause fear or other unpleasant feelings. By putting a cross on a continuum, the patient could mark the measure of his anxiety, that is the measure of his readiness to avoid the anxiety-evoking situation. We then calculated the median of each and every item. This resulted in obtaining two more or less identical groups as to size. One group which recorded relatively little and one group which recorded relatively a great deal of pain. The following day, that is, the day of the operation we again measured the pain. This time the procedure was as follows:

We recorded the subjective pain judgement the moment the patient asked for his first analgetic injection or if no injection was requested, 4 hours after the patient's arrival in the recovery room. We classified the patient's verbal report of his pain on the spot as follows:

0 = the patient states to have no pain
1 = the patient states he has very little pain
2 = the patient states he has moderate pain
3 = the patient states he has unbearable pain

The number of analgesic injections required by the patient within 10 hours after surgery was also used as a measure of pain. We equally noted the time which elapsed between arrival in the recovery room and the first request for an injection.

We furthermore employed a rating scale as developed by Chambers and Price (5) to qualify observed pain. Included was:

– the measure of the patient's attention to pain
– his worries about his state of health
– the measure of his mental strain
– the patient's expression of his pain
– the degree of his muscle tenseness
– his facial expression
– perspiration
– sounds made by the patient
– feeling of nausea.

The readings of the observation scale were as follows.

After a brief observation of the patient the instant he requested his first analgesic injection or otherwise four hours after his arrival in the recovery room, we recorded our impressions as regards each of the nine above mentioned items, on the linear scale. We then calculated the median score of each item separately. The two patient groupings thus obtained were practically identical as to their size: one group with relatively low and one group with relatively high pain scores.

With the exception of three, the pain scores revealed significant correlations. No significant correlation was found for factors relating to the time-interval between surgery and the first request for an analgesic injection, to perspiration and to the feeling of nausea. It can be assumed that these latter factors beside measuring pain give indications of other personality aspects as well.

Results of this study show a significant correlation at a 5% level between the degree of anxiety and the degree of pain. The group of patients reporting relatively severe pain was also the group with the highest anxiety score.

Anxiety is therefore considered to play a prominent role in the individual differences in pain felt by patients with similar surgical operations The number of narcotic injections administered 10 hours after surgery shows a significant correlation at a 1% level with the severity of the pain as perceived by the patient himself. Thus it is imperative that efforts directed toward effective reduction of pain should take into account the fact that the patient's perception of pain will be considerably influenced by his feelings of anxiety.

REFERENCES

1. Tursky, B. & O'Connell, D., Reliability and interjudgement. Predictability of subjective judgements of electrocutaneous stimulation. *Psychophysiology* 9, 3 (1972).
2. Beecher, H. K., *Measurement of subjective responses: Quantitative effects of drugs.* Oxford University Press, New York 1959.
3. Parbrook, G. D., Steel, D. F. & Dalrymple, D. G., Factors predisposing to postoperative pain and pulmonary complications. *Brit. J. Anaesth.* 45, 21 (1973).
4. Eikenbroek, H. J. & Herzberg, P. G. J. A., Over het verband tussen preoperatieve angst en postoperatieve pijn. Unpublished observations.
5. Chambers, W. G. & Price, G. G., Influence of nurse upon effects of analgesics administered. *Nursing Research* 16, 3 (1967).

THE MEASUREMENT OF PAIN:

THE CLINICAL PHARMACOLOGIST

H. MATTIE

Ages before pharmacology became a distinct branch of science, one of the most potent analgesics of today was already used in clinical practise: that was morphine, albeit as a component of opium, and not in its pure form. Another potent analgesics has also been known for many years: aspirin, which was used as an analgesic, and as an anti-inflammatory drug, long before formal standards for the conduct of clinical trials were invented to establish the efficacy of drugs. The reason I want to remind you of these well known facts is to warn you not to dismiss lightly this so called 'clinical experience'. On the other hand, we all know of remedies in which generations of doctors believed, that have now been proven to be worthless. Therefore, we really need some standards to establish the efficacy of drugs in general, and of analgesic drugs particularly. From clinical experience it was well known that morphine had a different mode of action from salicylates. Salicylic acid was found in the search for an alternative to quinine as an antipyretic drug. Where quinine comes from peruvian bark, salicylic acid was derived from willow bark; its analgesic and anti-inflammatory properties were only discovered later.

When pharmacologists began to study analgesics, they tried to invent animal tests to measure the effect of analgesics on pain. This has proven to be not very easy: in the first place because it is difficult to define animal pain, apart from the difficulty in defining pain at all. The reasoning, however, behind all animal tests is, that in human behaviour, the sensation of pain is coupled to more or less adequate reactions to harmful stimuli; now, in animals the same sort of harmful stimuli provoke reactions that are apparently also adequate. It can be stated, that all animal tests to detect analgesic properties in a drug, are tests in which inhibition of those seemingly adequate stimuli can be demonstrated. Pharmacologists who choose their words

59

carefully, therefore do not speak of pain reactions, but of nociceptive reactions. On the whole, this kind of test has indeed been proven to be very useful in the screening of new drugs for analgetic properties, but nevertheless they are black boxes: something is going into it, something is coming out, but nobody knows what the animal feels, and feeling is what matters, speaking of pain. One obvious example of the uncoupling of nociceptive stimuli from pain is familiar to anaesthetists: a lightly anaesthetized patient will still react to nociceptive stimuli adequately, while we assume he does not feel pain; the reaction of the patient can even be more forceful than normal, and may be compared with the so-called sham rage after stimulation in decerebrate animals.

Animal tests can be divided roughly in two classes. In the first place we have tests like the hot plate test, the writhing test and the tail flick test. In the hot plate tests mice are placed on a hot plate and within a short time they start licking their paws. This makes sense. The writhing test is done by injecting an irritating substance intraperitoneally in mice, on which they start, for one reason or another, to rub their bellies against the surface they are placed upon. In the tail flick test the tail of the animal is heated by a lamp and, as may be expected, the tail is swept away from the lamp. What is measured in all these tests is the time between stimulus and reaction. All these reactions are inhibited by morphine, and these tests are also very useful in discovering drugs with morphine-like action. Moreover, they make it possible to measure the relative potency of these drugs rather accurately. The interesting thing is that aspirin might not have been discovered in this way, because aspirin and other antipyretic analgesics behave very poorly in this kind of tests. It is much easier to detect the anti-inflammatory properties of those drugs. Most often this is done by measuring the degree of inhibition of oedema formation in the hind paw of a rat, after local injection of an irritating substance, e.g. carrageenin. From this a second class of nociceptive tests has been derived: an inflamed paw as just described, is pinched, a reaction is evoked, a sqeak or something. This kind of nociceptive reaction is indeed inhibited by antipyretic analgesics like aspirin. It may be stated that all modern analgetic drugs have been developed by employing tests like those described. However, for many other drugs, that are not regarded as analgesics it has been found in clinical practice that they are useful in the treatment of pain.

Many investigators have tried to elucidate the analgesic actions of drugs in experimental pain in man.

By techniques, that were nearly forgotten since the days of the Inquisition, human volunteers are made to suffer pain. One problem in this kind of experiments is of course, the choice of subjects. One would prefer an unbiased sample of the population, but one might argue whether anybody who voluntarily undergoes the infliction of pain, may be called a 'normal healthy volunteer'. This may be one reason why extrapolation from this kind of experiments to the clinical situation is rather hazardous. The advantage of human studies is that two qualities can be measured, namely pain threshold and pain tolerance, or suprathreshold. Moreover, these are both expressions of pain, and not mere reactions.

Very well known is the so-called tourniquet pain, or ischemic pain. The cuff of an ordinary blood pressure manometer is fastened to the upper arm. The arm is drained of venous blood, for instance by raising the arm, and the cuff is inflated to 250 mm Hg. The subject can tell the investigator when he begins to feel pain, and when pain becomes unbearable. At that point a good clinical investigator deflates the cuff. Another test is the applying of pressure to the Achilles tendon. This has the advantage that the pressure can be measured accurately. The development of many variations is due to the fact that none of them is really satisfactory. Again it is interesting to note that the morphine-like drugs are efficient in this kind of test, while aspirin-like drugs often give conflicting results. A very interesting study in this context is that of Bloomfield & Hurwitz (1). They studied their modification of the tourniquet experiments in volunteers, that is, laboratory technicians and the like, with aspirin. In a double blind study aspirin showed to be significantly more potent than a placebo for the pain threshold, while the difference for the pain tolerance was not so impressive. Then they undertook to study aspirin in patients with post-episiotomy pain, again double blind in comparison with placebo, and the drug showed to be effective. Now, in the same patients who were in the episiotomy experiment they studied the tourniquet pain. To their dismay there was no correlation at all between the effect of aspirin in the test and in clinical pain. This indicates, what was felt intuitively by many doctors, that human laboratory pain is something different than clinical pain. It is even conceivable that clinical pain itself is no distinct entity. It seems to me that postoperative pain, which is so often used to establish the effect of drugs, is very much different from pain in rheumatoid arthritis, or pain from malignant disease. In the latter, the whole state of mind of the patient will be very different from that in a patient that just has been relieved from an inflamed appendix, or a myoma.

In conclusion, animal pharmacology and clinical pharmacology are very important for our understanding of these drugs; but there is no substitute for careful clinical observation of every patient.

REFERENCE

1. Bloomfield, S. S. & Hurwitz, H. N., Tourniquet and episiotomy pain as test models for aspirin-like analgetics. *J. Clin. Pharmac.*, *10*, 361 (1970).

PART TWO

MEASUREMENT OF RESPIRATORY
AND ANAESTHETIC GASES

IN VIVO AND IN VITRO MEASUREMENT OF BLOOD pH – PCO$_2$ – PO$_2$

M. K. SYKES

The in vitro measurement of blood-gas tensions or pH takes several minutes even when the apparatus has been previously calibrated. If the apparatus has to be prepared for use or the sample transmitted to a remote laboratory for analysis, the result may not be available for thirty minutes or more. In a rapidly changing clinical situation such a delay may prejudice a patient's chance of survival. For this reason many workers have turned their attention to the possibility of in vivo measurements. Unhappily, many of the problems are still unsolved and many clinicians have therefore moved towards the provision of semi- or completely automated equipment for in vitro measurements in the hope that the rapid analysis of many samples can replace continuous in vivo analysis. These three approaches will now be discussed in more detail.

IN VIVO MEASUREMENTS
In vivo measurements are most simply performed in an exteriorised loop of the circulation, such as the circuit of a heart-lung machine or artificial kidney. In these circumstances the blood is heparinised and there is usually a large diameter conduit into which the electrode can be inserted. Repeated removal for recalibration is possible and the cuvette can be designed to minimize pressure and blood flow velocity artefacts and thus to secure optimal performance. These circumstances provide the best opportunities for overcoming the major problems inherent in the use of indwelling electrodes for thrombosis can be avoided, frequent recalibration can be performed and there is every opportunity to design the most suitable environment for the electrode. Despite these propitious considerations few centres use continuous monitoring routinely. It is not surprising, therefore, that even fewer workers have been prepared to tackle the problems associated with intravascular measurements. There is, however, one situation in which continuous intravascular monitoring of arterial PO$_2$ could be extremely valuable and

that is in the case of the neonate with acute respiratory failure. These babies suffer major rapid fluctuations of PO_2 and PCO_2 due to changes in ventilation or intrapulmonary shunt. It has been shown that hyperoxia for even a few hours may cause retrolental fibroplasia whilst longer periods of high oxygen concentration breathing may lead to chronic lung changes. The use of an oxygen transducer in the umbilical artery not only permits continuous monitoring of PO_2 but also obviates the need for repeated blood sampling with the resultant anaemia. Parker et al. (1) have described the construction and use of a silver-lead galvanic cell which is sealed into the end of a PTFE tube of 0.8 mm outside diameter. This has been used with some success in the neonate, but difficulties have arisen form protein deposition on the membrane. This has caused the output to fall off with time so that frequent recalibration is necessary.

A third method of in vivo measurement utilises the mass spectrometer for the analysis of a small gas sample which is obtained by diffusion through a membrane inserted into the blood stream. A plastic catheter with a thin membrane at its tip is inserted into the vessel and a small, continuous gas sample withdrawn from the catheter into the mass spectrometer. Rapid diffusion of gases is achieved by the use of a thin silicone membrane, thus permitting the continuous sampling of equilibrated gas. There are difficulties in calibrating the system in vivo but the system has great potential for the mass spectrometer can analyse a wide range of gases and the same principle can also be used for in vitro measurements (2, 3, 4.)

In view of the difficulties in maintaining an electrode in the circulation without the occurrence of thrombosis, other workers have turned their attention to measurements of blood-gases in tissue. Unfortunately, tissue measurements in the major organs such as the brain, heart, liver or kidney are difficult because the organs are relatively inaccessible. Tissue measurements in more superficial areas are greatly dependent on blood flow and the relationship between the measured tension in tissue and those existing at the mitochondria is not clearly defined (5, 6). For these reasons the interpretation of tissue measurements is difficult. Nevertheless, the ease with which tissue electrodes can be implanted and the freedom from thrombotic problems has led to a number of developments in this field. For example Strauss et al. (7) have designed a bare wire electrode which is threaded through the ear lobe whilst Kwan & Fatt (8) have developed an electrode which can be applied to the surface of the conjunctiva. Surface electrodes are easy to dislodge, however, and at the present time it appears that tissue monitoring does not have very much to recommend it.

IN VITRO MEASUREMENTS

Most of the apparatus in use today has been designed for use with capillary blood samples, the volume of blood required varying from 120-400 ml. In order to measure PO$_2$, PCO$_2$ and pH on such small samples a common cuvette is required. The taking and handling of capillary samples presents many problems, and their analysis even more. It is not surprising, therefore, that a high degree of technical skill is required to achieve satisfactory results. The use of larger samples of arterial blood overcomes most of the problems of sample handling but there are still many sources of error which can lead to inaccurate results. Since few workers regularly duplicate their analyses on two sets of equipment or use tonometered blood samples to check their apparatus, these errors are usually not recognised. For clinical purposes, small errors may be acceptable. However, on many occasions over the past thirteen years, we have observed errors of up to 10 mm Hg PCO$_2$, 20 mm Hg PO$_2$ and 0.2 units pH when analysing blood samples on apparatus which has been correctly calibrated with standard buffers or gases and which was apparently functioning normally. These errors were detected by comparison of blood samples on duplicate machines and by regular checking with tonometered blood samples.

PO$_2$

The development of the oxygen electrode has been well described by Lübbers (9), most workers now using the Clark type of electrode. Although the use of small-diameter platinum electrodes has obviated the need to stir the blood most commercial electrodes still give a lower reading with a blood sample than with a gas of the same tension. The value of this blood-gas difference varies with each electrode and from day to day but usually amounts to 2 to 6 per cent of the reading. For accurate work the blood-gas difference must be determined each day by measuring the PO$_2$ of blood or liquid samples of known PO$_2$. This can be accomplished by equilibrating the blood-sample in a tonometer such as that described by Adams and Morgan-Hughes (10). The methods of calibration, sources of error and problems associated with the use of oxygen electrodes have been detailed elsewhere (11). However, it is particularly important to ensure that the membrane is intact, that there are no air bubbles under the membrane or in the cuvette when the reading is taken, and that the electrode responds rapidly and is linear throughout the range of use. With great care an accuracy of $\pm$ 2 mm Hg ($\pm$ SD) can be achieved in the 0 – 150 mm range. The errors become much greater in the higher ranges due to the restricted scale length on most commercial meters and to the rapid reduction in PO_2 resulting from the consumption of oxygen by leucocytes. Errors also arise from the presence of volatile anaesthetic agents (12).

PCO_2

Although PCO_2 can be determined by interpolation (as in the Astrup technique) most commercial blood-gas analysers now incorporate a CO_2 electrode for measurement of PCO_2. This is basically a pH electrode which measures the change in pH of a bicarbonate solution trapped in a mesh between the membrane and the electrode surface. The response is logarithmic so that the greatest accuracy is obtained at low PCO_2 values. The response is slower than that of an oxygen electrode and errors are usually due to a failure to achieve equilibrium between the PCO_2 in the blood and bicarbonate solution. Errors are minimised by ensuring that the membrane is intact, that the response is not sluggish and by using a reference gas with a PCO_2 close to that expected in the blood sample (13, 14, 15).

pH

Most pH electrodes now utilise the capillary type of electrode with a calomel reference electrode (16). Electrodes which read accurately when tested with buffers may read inaccurately when blood is inserted. Accuracy can only be maintained by comparing the reading on a second electrode system or by using a stabilised serum preparation as a control (17).

SEMI-AUTOMATED APPARATUS FOR PO_2, PCO_2 AND pH

During the past five years semi-automatic blood-gas analysis equipment has become available. This equipment programmes the calibration, wash, and sample sequences, which are therefore carried out in a repeatable fashion for each blood sample. This enhances accuracy. However, the use of a preset time for display of the readings presupposes that all the electrodes are responding briskly and that they have reached final values within the time allowed. Since these machines are designed to accept capillary samples the cuvette volume is kept small by incorporating two or three of the electrodes in a common cuvette. This, and the added complexity of the apparatus, renders breakdowns more catastrophic when they do occur. The behaviour of one of these automatic machines has recently been evaluated against several of the older manual types of apparatus and shown to compare favourably (18). Another model not only provides a digital readout of PO_2, PCO_2 and pH but automatically computes base excess, total CO_2 and HCO_3

as well. Experience of the use of these analysers in hospital practice suggests that they greatly increase the number of analyses that can be performed by a single operator. Operator fatigue is less and to that extent accuracy may be increased. It is also probable that relatively inexperienced operators may be able to work these machines. Although completely automated analysis is not yet with us, these machines represent a significant advance in blood-gas analysis.

APPARATUS FOR MEASUREMENT OF O$_2$ AND CO$_2$ CONTENT
The advent of the O$_2$ electrode removed the need to calculate PO$_2$ from oxygen content or saturation and although the latter measurements are not strictly within the scope of this review, recent developments deserve a mention. Although the Van Slyke apparatus is still the standard by which other methods are judged, the method is slow and great technical skill is required to achieve consistent results. Developments in electrode technology led to the evolution of a number of methods for measuring O$_2$ and CO$_2$ content which were based on the change in tensions observed when these gases are driven out of the blood into solution (19). More recently semi-automated equipment has become avialable for measurement of Hb, HbCO and oxygen saturation or for the direct measurement of O$_2$ content. The analyses are quick, relatively easy to perform but calibration against the Van Slyke has not always been reported to yield satisfactory results. Nevertheless, developments in this field are of interest to those workers who are interested in measuring shifts in the dissociation curve, intrapulmonary shunts or cardiac output by the Fick method.

SAMPLE HANDLING
It is perhaps important to stress once again that the analysis can only be accurate if the blood sample is correctly taken, stored and then thoroughly mixed before insertion into the analyser. The mixing is particularly important when small samples are being used for the measurement of O$_2$ content for rapid settling of the red cells can easily lead to errors in content measurement of 3 - 5 volumes per cent. Arterialised venous samples can be used for PCO$_2$ or pH measurement but not for PO$_2$ whilst capillary samples can be used for all three measurements providing the patient is not shocked and full vasodilatation has been achieved (11). Arterial samples are always preferable if they can be obtained without disturbing the patient's steady state but they should always be taken into glass syringes if the arterial PO$_2$ is above normal levels (20).

CONCLUSION

Determinations of PO_2, PCO_2 and pH are still subject to major errors which may be severe enough to lead to mistakes in diagnosis and treatment. Intravascular electrodes are not yet satisfactory and have a limited sphere of use. The advent of semi-automated analysers will probably increase the accuracy of measurements made by relatively unskilled personnel but experience in their use is still limited. The regular testing of electrode systems by known blood or plasma samples is essential for the maintenance of accuracy of measurement.

REFERENCES

1. Parker, D., Key, A., Davies, R., Scopes, J. W. & Marcovitch, H., A disposable catheter tip transducer for continuous measurement of blood oxygen tension in vivo. *Bio-Med. Engn.* 6, 313 (1971).
2. Woldring, S., Owens, G. & Woolford, D. C., Blood-gases: continuous in vivo recording of partial pressures by mass spectrography. *Science* 153, 885 (1966).
3. Wald, A., Hass, W. K., Siew, F. P. & Wood, D. H., Continuous measurement of blood-gases *in vivo* by mass spectroscopy. *Med. biol. Eng.* 8, 111 (1970).
4. Brantigan, J. W., Gott, V. L. & Martz, M. N., Teflon membrane for measurement of blood and intramyocardial gas tensions by mass spectroscopy. *J. appl. Physiol.* 32, 276 (1972).
5. Silver, I. A., The measurement of oxygen tension in tissues. In: Payne, J. P. & Hill, D. W. (ed.), *A symposium on oxygen measurements in blood and tissues and their significance.* J. & A. Churchill, London 1966.
6. Cater, D. B., The significance of oxygen tension measurements in tissues. In: Payne, J. P. & Hill, D. W. (ed.), *A symposium on oxygen measurements in blood and tissues and their significance.* J. & A. Churchill, London 1966.
7. Strauss, J., Beran, A. V. & Baker, R., Continuous O_2 monitoring of newborn and older infants and of children. *J. appl. Physiol.* 33, 238 (1972).
8. Kwan, M. & Fatt, I., A noninvasive method of continuous arterial oxygen tension estimation from measured palpebral conjunctival oxygen tension. *Anaesthesiology* 35, 309 (1971).
9. Lübbers, D. W., Methods of measuring oxygen tensions of blood and organ surfaces. In: Payne, J. P. & Hill, D. W. (ed.), *A symposium on oxygen measurements in blood and tissues and their significance.* J. & A. Churchill, London (1966).
10. Adams, A. P. & Morgan-Hughes, J. O., Determination of the blood-gas factor of the oxygen electrode using a new tonometer. *Brit. J. Anaesth.* 39, 107 (1967).
11. Adams, A. P., Morgan–Hughes, J. O. & Sykes, M. K., pH and blood-gas analysis. Methods of measurement and sources of error using electrode systems, Part 1. *Anaesthesia* 22, 575 (1967).
12. Severinghaus, J. W., Weiskopf, R. B., Nishimura, M. & Bradley, A. F., Oxygen electrode errors due to polarographic reduction of halothane. *J. appl. Physiol.* 31, 640 (1971).
13. Adams, A. P., Morgan–Hughes, J. O. & Sykes, M. K., pH and blood-gas analysis. Part 2. Measurement of carbon dioxide tension and acid-base. *Anaesthesia* 23, 47 (1968).

14. Severinghaus, J. W., Measurements of blood gases: PO_2 and PCO_2. *Ann. New York Acad. Sci.* 148, 115 (1968).
15. Lunn, J. N. & Mapleson, W. W., The Severinghaus CO_2 electrode: a theoretical and experimental assessment. *Brit. J. Anaesth.* 35, 666 (1963).
16. Sykes, M. K., The determination of pH. In: Scurr, C. F., and Feldman, S. A. (eds.) *Scientific Foundations of Anaesthesia.* Heinemann, London (1970).
17. Bird, B. D. & Henderson, F. A., The use of serum as a control in acid-base determination. *Brit. J. Anaesth.* 43, 592 (1971).
18. Hill, D. W. & Tilsley, C., A comparative study of the performance of five commercial blood-gas and pH electrode analysers. *Brit. J. Anaesth.* 45, 647 (1973).
19. Solymar, M., Rucklidge, M. A. & Prys–Roberts, C., A modified approach to the polarographic measurement of blood O_2 content. *J. appl. Physiol.* 30, 272 (1971).
20. Scott, P. V., Horton, J. N. & Mapleson, W. W., Leakage of oxygen from blood and water samples stored in plastic and glass syringes. *Brit. Med. J.* 3, 512 (1971).

THE MEASUREMENT OF OXYGEN IN THE GAS PHASE

JULIAN M. LEIGH

Many physical methods lend themselves to the analysis of oxygen in the gas phase. All these must be standardised against chemical/volumetric methods which are *absolute*, i.e. requiring no calibration. In the latter, oxygen is absorbed in a burette system, usually by alkaline pyrogallol, and measurements of volume change at constant pressure give the quantity of oxygen gas present in the original sample. (Carbon dioxide must be absorbed by KOH or NaOH *prior to* the oxygen absorption.)

POLAROGRAPHY

The polarographic electrode, in which the current resulting from the reduction of molecules of oxygen at a platinum cathode is a direct function of Po_2, has already been described by Professor Sykes in an earlier chapter. The same device that is used for blood Po_2 measurements can also be used to measure oxygen in the gas phase. Several detectors of this type have also been manufactured for monitoring oxygen in anaesthetic circuits, incubators, etc. – e.g. the I.M.I. oxygen monitor (Becton, Dickinson Ltd.).

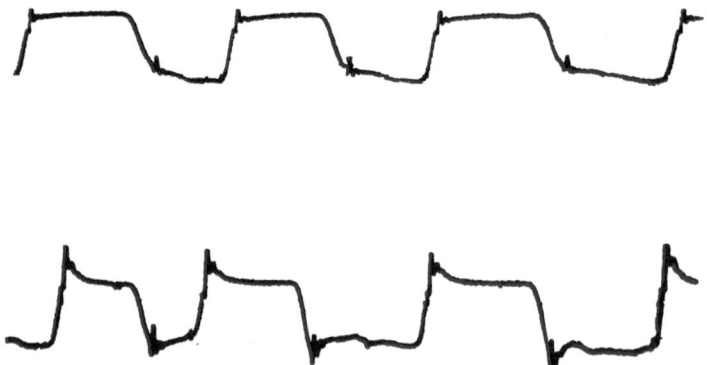

Fig. 1. Tidal oxygen at two damping settings of the 'RESPONSE' potentiometer on the Beckman OM 11. Compare with upper trace in Fig. 4.

These polarographic electrodes usually have a slow response time, and therefore cannot follow tidal changes in oxygen concentration. Beckman have recently introduced a rapid response polarographic analyser, the O.M. 11, with a draw through head similar in external appearance to their well established infra-red carbon dioxide analyser. This device is fitted with a 'RESPONSE' potentiometer which enables the user to adjust the damping of the output signal (Fig. 1).

GALVANIC FUEL CELL

In a galvanic fuel cell the oxidation of a fuel is utilised to produce a voltage. Several experimental fuel cells have been produced in which the measured voltage is used to determine an unknown oxygen concentration. A practical system which is commercially available and which is capable of following tidal changes in oxygen concentration is the zirconium oxide fuel cell produced by Westinghouse (Fig. 2). Essentially the detector consists of a cylindrical battery with porous platinum electrodes. The outside is in contact with a reference oxygen concentration (usually air) and the inside is in contact with the gas sample as it is pumped through. At any time, the voltage difference from the inside to the outside of the battery is related to the logarithm of the oxygen concentration gradient. Unfortunately, this system functions at a temperature of 850 °C, at which many anaesthetic agents are oxidised and consequently interfere with measurements causing low readings.

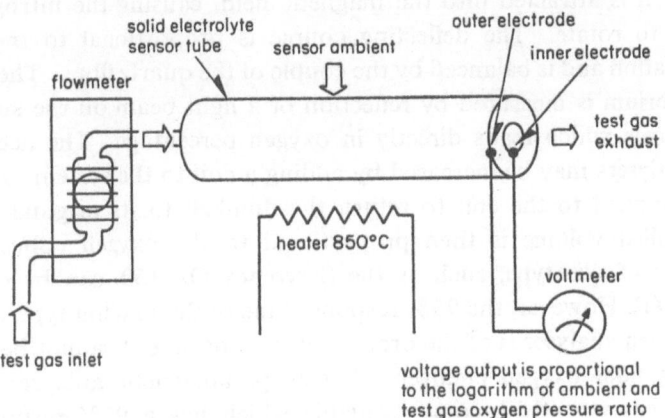

Fig. 2. The zirconium oxide galvanic fuel cell – Westinghouse.

PARAMAGNETIC SUSCEPTIBILITY

Oxygen is paramagnetic, in other words it tends to align itself in the lines of flux in a magnetic field. Nitrogen is diamagnetic, i.e. its susceptibility to magnetisation is negative and it tends to be repelled form a magnetic field.

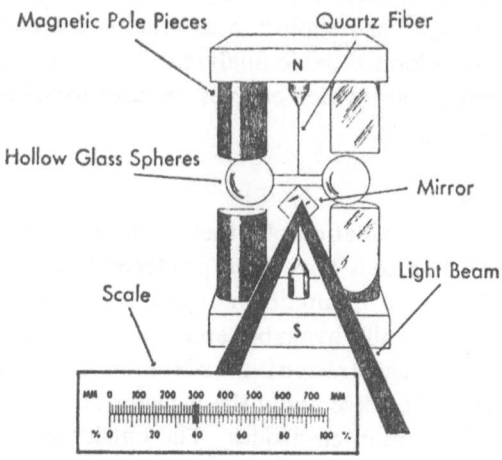

Fig. 3. Pauling-type paramagnetic oxygen analyser.

In a Pauling-type paramagnetic oxygen analyser (Fig. 3), a small nitrogen filled glass dumbell is suspended on a quartz fibre in an eccentric permanent magnetic field. If the oxygen concentration in the analyser is increased, then the oxygen is attracted into the magnetic field, causing the nitrogen filled dumbell to rotate. The deflecting couple is proportional to the oxygen concentration and is balanced by the couple of the quartz fibre. The position at equilibrium is measured by reflection of a light beam on the suspension onto a scale which reads directly in oxygen percentage. The accuracy of these analysers may be increased by adding a coil to the system. A voltage can be applied to the coil to return the dumbell to its original position. This applied voltage is then proportional to the oxygen concentration. Analysers of this type, such as the Servomex OA.150, can be extremely accurate (1). However, the 95% response time of the Pauling-type paramagnetic oxygen analyser is of the order of 9 seconds, and it cannot be used for following tidal oxygen changes. A new paramagnetic analyser (Rapox, Godart) has recently become available which has a 95% response time comparable with that of infra-red carbon dioxide analysers (2) (Fig. 4). The measuring principle of this analyser is that of a pneumatic Wheatstone bridge. A pump PI (Fig. 5) draws the sample gas and a reference gas into their respective sample chambers. A second pump P2 draws these gases at

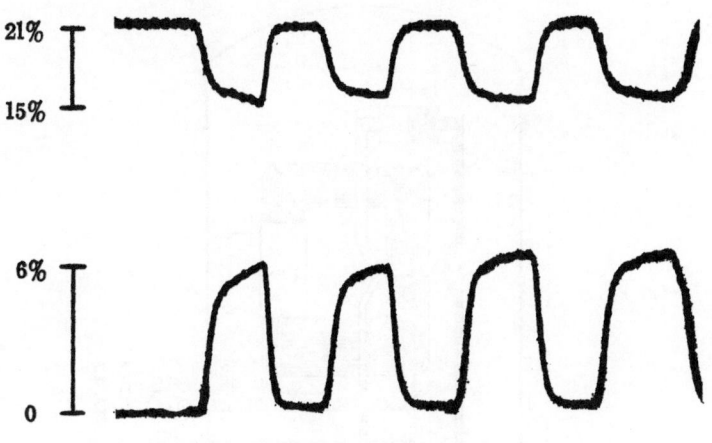

Air Breathing

Fig. 4. Tidal O_2 and CO_2 during air breathing. The latter by an infra-red analyser and the former by the Rapox.

a constant rate via a T-junction set within an electro-magnetic field. Thus the reference gas, usually air, is applied to one limb of the T-piece and the sample gas to the other limb. The resistance to gas flow in each limb will be increased if that gas is paramagnetic and susceptible to the influence of the magnetic field. Under conditions of constant flow, this change in resistance will be reflected by a proportional change in pressure across the limbs of the T-piece. This pressure difference is sensed by a differential capacitative pressure transducer. The accuracy and stability of the instrument is improved by modulating the magnetic field at a frequency of 25 Hz and sampling the pressure change at a similar frequency. Unfortunately this analyser cannot be used during intermittent positive pressure ventilation as pressure changes produce false deflections in the transducer system for which there is no simple method of compensation.

GAS CHROMATOGRAPHY
The theory of this general purpose analytical technique is described in detail in the chapter by Dr. Burm and his colleagues. In essence, when a gaseous mixture is passed in a carrier gas stream through a column, then the components will be delayed according to their affinity for a stationary phase within the column. The emergence of the separated substances is sensed and transduced into an electrical signal by an appropriate detector such as a katharometer.

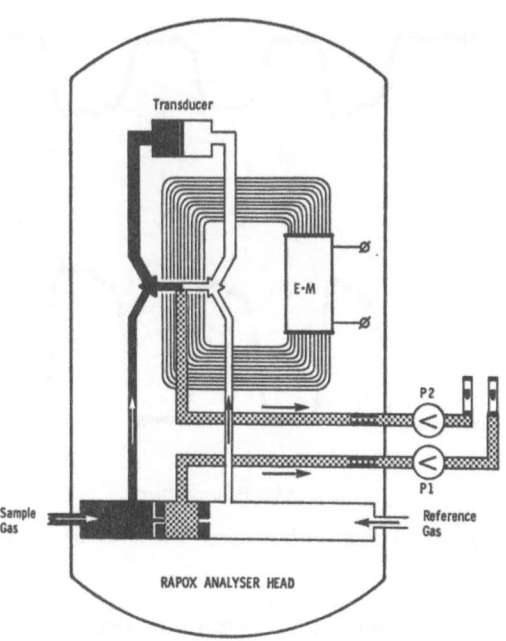

Fig. 5. Analyser head of the Rapox oxygen analyser – Godart.

A practical system for measuring oxygen by gas chromatography usually involves a simultaneous carbon dioxide measurement and may also include, in the context of anaesthesia, the detection and separation of nitrous oxide. This is achieved by running two chromatographic columns in parallel at room temperature. A column packed with 'Poropak' achieves the separation of carbon dioxide and nitrous oxide, while a column filled with artificial zeolite (molecular sieve) will separate oxygen from nitrogen. Detection is achieved with a thermal conductivity detector (katharometer). The chromatogram is written out by a potentiometric recorder and the peak areas are proportional to the concentrations of the individual gases.

The advantage of gas chromatography is that it is a very sensitive technique, i.e. a large electrical signal can be produced from microlitre samples. A disadvantage is that it is slow and cannot be used for tidal oxygen recordings.

MASS SPECTROMETRY

Mass spectrometry offers both high sensitivity and a frequency response capable of following tidal changes in gas concentration. All substances have mass and, when ionised, a mass to charge ratio, and it is the detection of this which forms the operating principle of mass spectrometers. Sample gas is sucked into the mass spectrometer via a fine metal catheter. Part of this gas enters the mass spectrometer proper through a molecular leak. The sample is ionised by bombardment with electrons and, in a *magnetic mass spectrometer* (Fig. 6), the charged particles are accelerated within a magnetic field. Because of the nature of the magnetic field the ions with less mass attain an orbit of lesser diameter than those with a greater mass. The accelerating voltage is constantly varied from zero upwards and, as a result, each separate mass beam is focused serially on the collector. The collector current is proportional to the number of ions arriving at any instant in time.

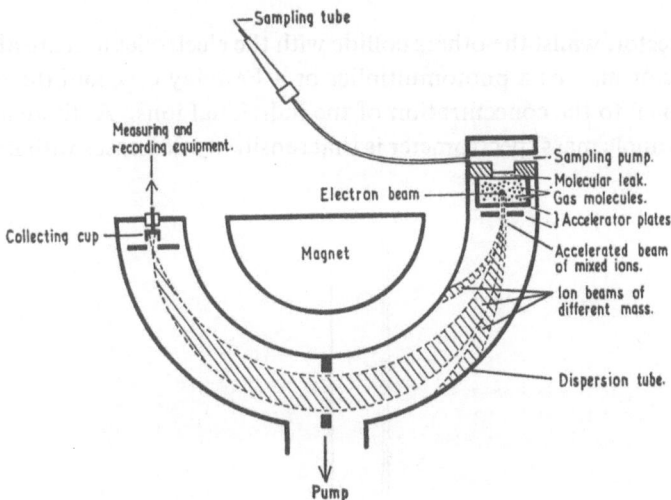

Fig. 6. Magnetic mass spectrometer.

The ions are separated by a different method in a quadrupole mass spectrometer (Fig. 7). This type of mass spectrometer is very much smaller and consists of four electrodes with opposite pairs connected together. Two signals are applied to the electrodes. First, an RF signal of gradually increasing amplitude and 180° out of phase on each pair of electrodes. Secondly, a DC ramp from zero volts to a set value (which governs the highest mass detectable) which is superimposed on the RF signal and one pair of electrodes receives a negative voltage whilst the other pair receives a positive voltage. The resulting field is hyperbolic and the ions corkscrew their way towards the detector. At any instant only ions of a specific mass/charge ratio arrive

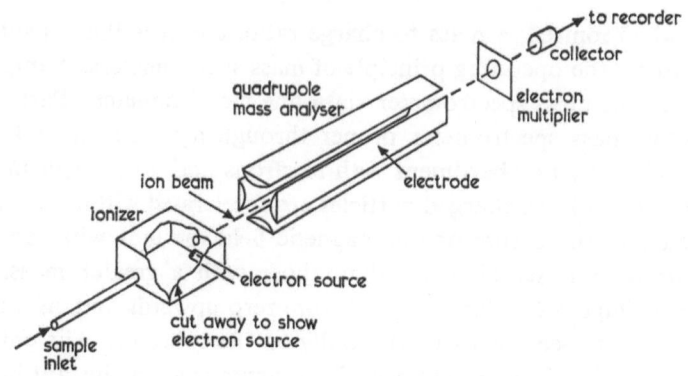

Fig. 7. Quadrupole mass spectrometer.

at the detector, whilst the others collide with the electrodes and are absorbed. The detector may be a photomultiplier or a Faraday cup, and the output is proportional to the concentration of the individual ions. A disadvantage of the quadrupole mass spectrometer is that sensitivity decreases with increasing mass.

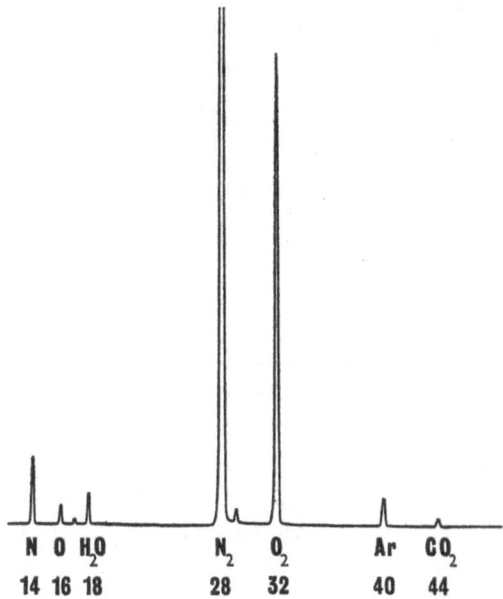

Fig. 8. Air spectrum – quadrupole mass spectrometer. The unlabelled peaks are OH at mass 17 and N_2H at mass 29.

For display, mass number is presented on the x axis and the processed detector signal on the *y* axis. The result is a spectrogram similar to that produced by gas chromatograph with peak areas proportional to the quantities of the different ions. The *x* axis may be swept at speeds varying from minutes to milliseconds. In the latter case, the display may only be presented on an oscilliscope and in the former is more usefully displayed on a potentiometric recorder for quantitative work.

An important difference from gas chromatography is that in mass spectrography the substances undergo 'cracking' into different ions. However, each substance has a characteristic cracking pattern with a maximal or 'base peak' and subsidiary peaks which always provide a 'finger-print' of the given substance. Fig. 8 shows the cracking pattern of air. It can be seen that oxygen has a base peak at mass 32, but some also appear at mass 16. When several substances are present the solution of simultaneous equations by on-line digital computation may be required to facilitate the analysis.

Since the DC voltage can be changed rapidly, alterations in the heights of individual peaks in the spectrum can be followed virtually continuously using 'peak followers' so the concentrations of various substances presen in the gas mixture can be displayed against time. Fig. 9 shows tidal oxygen (above) and tidal carbon dioxide (below) obtained on a quadrupole mass spectrometer used in the above manner.

With mass spectrometers in general, water vapour causes a problem. Unless

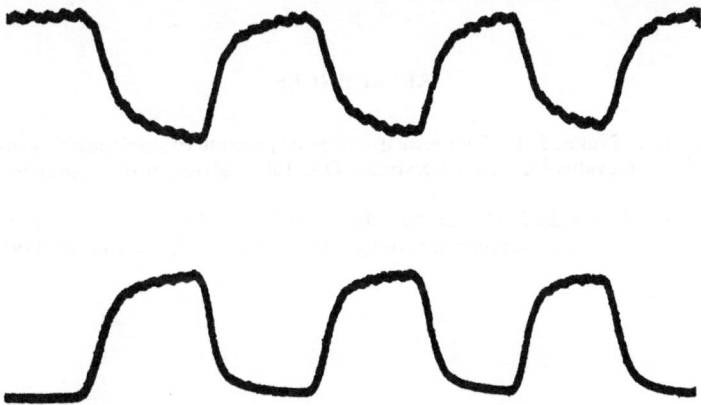

Fig. 9. Tidal O_2 (above) and tidal CO_2 (below) using a quadrupole mass spectrometer in the peak following mode.

the metal catheter is heated, especially at its tip, water vapour elutes in the same way as in a gas chromatograph. Fig. 10 shows tidal carbon dioxide (below) and tidal water (above). Both phase and amplitude distortion are quite clearly shown.

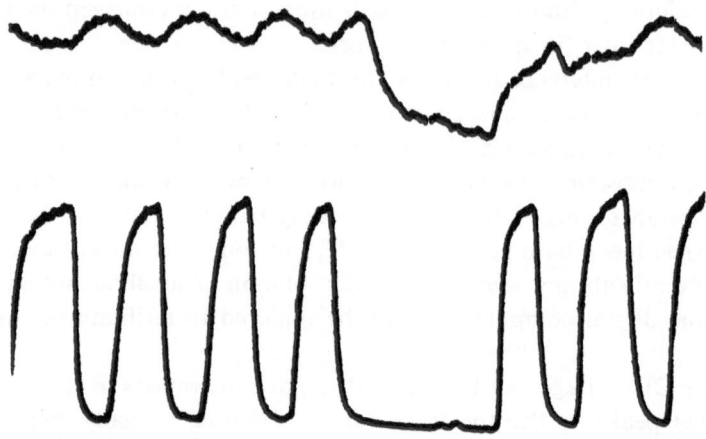

Fig. 10. Tidal H_2O (above) and CO_2 (below) – quadrupole mass spectrometer with imperfectly heated sampling probe. Both phase and amplitude distortion are shown due to the elution of the H_2O vapour in the system.

Mass spectrometers require careful maintenance, however, potentially they hold great promise, not only for accurate measurements of oxygen, but also for *any* substance which can be obtained in the gas phase.

REFERENCES

1. Ellis, F. R. & Nunn, J. F., The measurement of gaseous oxygen tension using paramagnetism: an evaluation of the Servomex OA. 150 analyser. *Brit. J. Anaesth.* 40, 569 (1968).
2. Conway, C. M., Leigh, J. M., Lindop, M. J. & Webb, D. A., An evaluation of the 'Rapox' rapid response paramagnetic oxygen analyser. *Brit. J. Anaesth.* 45, 1191 (1973).

CAPNOGRAPHY

P. J. JANSSEN

INTRODUCTION

After the work of Digby Leigh et al. (1) (2) in cardio-anaesthesia, of Burton (3) and others in general anaesthesia, and of Smalhout (4) in neuro-anaesthesia, the capnograph has become a familiar instrument to the anaesthetist. It is largely the purpose of this communication to sound a warning against the possibilities of incorrect interpretation of end-expiratory CO_2-percentages in relation to $PaCO_2$ values. Assumption of a constant interrelationship may easily lead to wrong conclusions and thence to wrong 'therapeutic' actions.

THE CAPNOGRAPH

A frequently used instrument is the Godart capnograph. It consists of an analyzer – the 'detector-head' – an amplifier, a suction pump, and a paper writer – the 'Omniascriptor' –.

The 'detector-head' of the complete capnograph system is of the Luft type (5). Its measuring principle is based on the fact that gases with dissimilar atoms readily absorb infra-red rays at a particular wavelength.

The analyzer contains two chambers, a reference chamber and a measuring chamber through which identical rays are passed from an infrared source. Beyond these chambers are two heat-sensitive detector cells. These are in direct contact but separated from each other by an thin metal diaphragm; close to this diaphragm another thin metal plate is mounted. These form a variable capacitor, or condenser microphone system.

The degree of the displacement of the thin metal diaphragm reflects relative expansion due to relative heating and relative absorption of infrared light by the relative concentrations of carbon dioxide in the reference and measuring chambers.

Directly after the infrared source the beams are interrupted at a rate of 25 per second by a chopper. By this mechanism an alternating current is generated in the detector cell. After amplification this signal current is displayed on an amperemeter dial. The meter is made specific for carbon dioxide by setting its maximal sensitivity at the band of maximum infrared absorbtion of carbon dioxide. The signal may also be recorded on a paper strip, resulting in a 'capnogram' (Fig. 1). The curve on this capnogram reflects the continuous changes in the carbon dioxide content of the ventilatory gases, and therefore this content may be measured at any given moment of the ventilatory cycle. Clinically the inspiratory and end-expiratory values of the CO_2-content are the most important.

BIOLOGICAL COMPONENTS INFLUENCING THE CAPNOGRAM

After carbon dioxide is generated within the cells of the tissues as one end-product of the Krebs' cycle it is transported by the circulating blood to the lung capillaries from where it diffuses into the lung alveoli; the organism then disposes of it by the mechanism of ventilation. From this it may be concluded that at least three factors may influence the ultimate capnograph readings. These are:

1. the metabolic rate of the tissues;
2. the state of the circulatory system;
3. the state of the ventilatory system,

at any given moment; these systems may naturally interact in both a positive and negative sense. A positive influence of one system thus may cancel a negative one of another, with a resultant absence of net change in the ultimate capnograph reading.

This important fact should be well kept in mind. Only by keeping two systems constant can one use the capnogram to evaluate and measure changes in the third system.

I.   *Changes in metabolic rate*

In normal clinical anaesthesia practice, changes in the over-all metabolic rate of the organism are usually slight, and are at least more or less constant. However, the influence of muscle relaxants on carbon dioxide production (body temperature) should not be underestimated, especially in air-conditioned operating-rooms.

Changes in this system never develop suddenly, except in cases of acute malignant hyperthermia or induced central hypothermia with the aid of extracorporeal circulation, where they arise acutely, and in cases of induced surface hypothermia, where they are brought about more slowly.

With altered carbon dioxide production, but unchanged carbon dioxide elimination in artificially ventilated patients, a deviation of normal $PaCO_2$ values is bound to follow.

II. *Changes in the circulatory state*

Metabolism remaining constant and total minute ventilation being correct for the artificially ventilated patients' condition, any lowering of the end-expiratory capnograph readings means that less carbon dioxide molecules are being offered to the lung alveoli for disposal to the outside air. This means that pulmonary perfusion, i.e. cardiac output, is reduced.

The capnogram may therefore give useful information of changes in cardiac output provided that ventilation remains constant (Fig. 2).

The capnograph readings will promptly follow changes in the circulatory state, be they acute or subacute. However, any acute lowering of these values always indicates a reduction of the cardiac output, provided the alveolar ventilation remains unaltered. In that case one should not attempt to normalize the capnogram values by reducing the alveolar ventilation, for in doing so the raised tissue PCO_2 resulting from reduced blood flow will be increased further. Appropriate measures should then be taken to restore the cardiac output.

Capnography may be of specific use in some heart operations, such as banding of the pulmonary artery in high pulmonary flow states, together with arterial blood gas values as reference (Fig. 3) (6).

III. *Changes in the ventilatory state*

It is necessary to attach the capnograph to the artificial ventilatory system as soon as the patient has been intubated. This will give us the initial end-expiratory carbon dioxide content of the ventilatory gases. The total minute ventilation is regulated in such a way that the end-expiratory capnogram value stays within 0.2% of the initial value. The actual PCO_2 is then determined in arterial or capillary blood in order to find the relationship between the $PaCO_2$ and the $F_{E'CO2}$.

This individual calibration of $F_{E'CO2}$ with $PaCO_2$ is necessary, as the relationship may vary in time, from patient to patient, and with the individual capnograph (Fig. 4).

With the aid of a simple nomogram the 'ideal' capnogram value corresponding with a $PaCO_2$ of 40 Torr may be determined (Fig. 5), – assuming that the circulatory and metabolic state have remained the same –.

Ventilation may then be adjusted as necessary to attain that ideal value during the rest of the operation either by slightly reducing alveolar ventil-

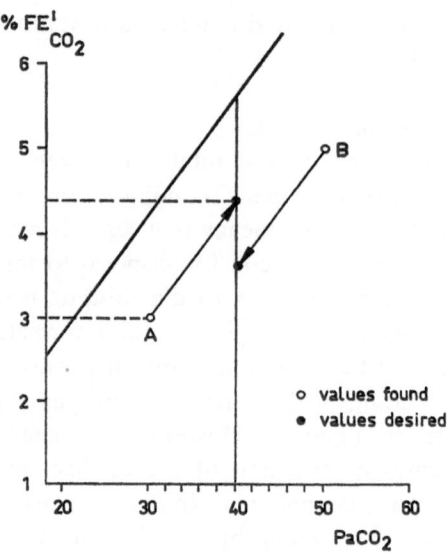

Fig. 5. The nomogram for determination of 'ideal $F_{E'CO_2}$ value'. On the abscissa the $PaCO_2$ in Torr; on the ordinate the $F_{E'CO_2}$ in % as measured on the capnograph CO_2 percentage scale. In patient A, a measured $PaCO_2$ of 30 Torr at a $F_{E'CO_2}$ of 3% means that ventilation has to be adjusted to attain a $F_{E'CO_2}$ of 4.4% in order to achieve a $PaCO_2$ of 40 Torr. Likewise the ventilation of patient B has to be adjusted so that a $F_{E'CO_2}$ of 3.6% is reached for a $PaCO_2$ of 40 Torr.
The remaining line on the graph represents a—E′CO_2 values assuming a zero a-E′CO_2 gradient.

ation and/or adding carbon dioxide to the ventilatory gas mixture(Fig. 6.)

In long operations it is wise to repeat the determination of acid-base and gas values. By measuring $F_{E'CO_2}$ continuously, the induced ventilatory component of acid-base balance may be much better kept in hand as one prevents gross hypo- or hyperventilation. In this respect it should be kept in mind that a ventilation induced change in $F_{E'CO_2}$ of 1% represents a change in $PaCO_2$ of close to 7 Torr; one percent reduction thus may mean a lowering of the $PaCO_2$ from an acceptable values of 36 Torr to a perhaps unacceptable level of about 29 Torr.

IV. *Special remarks on the per-operative use of the capnograph*
The necessity of 'calibrating' each individual patient with any individual capnograph has been mentioned already.
A capnographically determined $F_{E'CO_2}$ of 5% may mean a $PaCO_2$ of 40

Torr in one patient, whereas in another patient it may mean a $PaCO_2$ of 56 Torr (Fig. 7a and b).

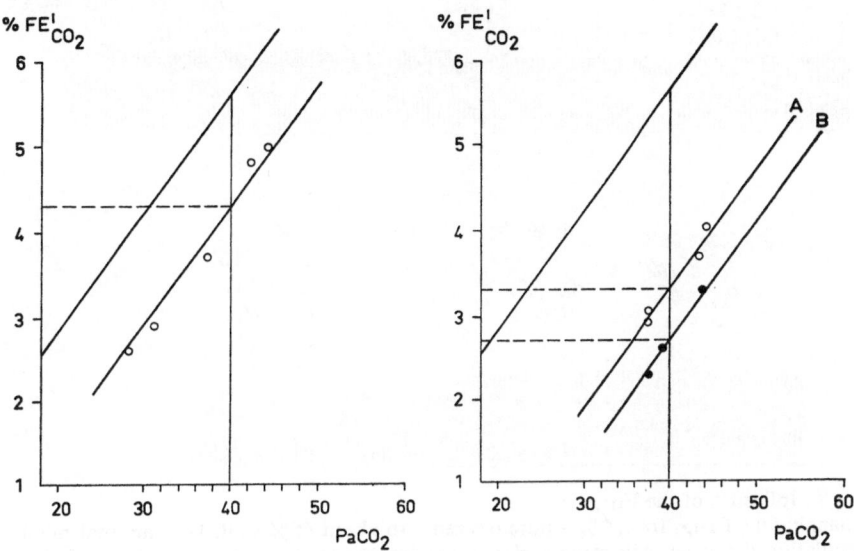

Fig. 7a. In this case a $F_{E'CO_2}$ of 4.3 % is necessary for a $PaCO_2$ of 40 Torr.

Fig. 7b. In the case of a circulation being basically changed by surgery – as in correction of several congenital heart defects – establishment of a 'new ideal $F_{E'CO_2}$ value' is necessary. In this patient a $F_{E'CO_2}$ of 2.7 % coincides with a $PaCO_2$ of 40 Torr before extracorporeal circulation (line B), whereas a value of 3.3 % was necessary after surgical correction (line A).
Both examples show that individual 'calibration' of the capnograph with $PaCO_2$ measurements is always indicated.

The end-expiratory capnogram value varies linearly with the percentage of nitrous oxide in the ventilatory gas mixture (Fig. 8). With a FI_{N_2O} of 70 % the end-expiratory capnograph value will be about one scale percentage higher than with a FI_{N_2O} of 0 % (pure oxygen) at the *same* $PaCO_2$ (7) as result of cross-sensitivity between the two gases (8).

Thus far the use of the capnogram as a continuous indicator of the $PaCO_2$ has been discussed.

However, the capnogram may also be used to great advantage by the anaesthetist as a general monitoring device. Some possibilities are:

a. a gradual increase in end-tidal capnogram values may indicate insufficient alveolar ventilation as well as exhaustion of soda lime absorbers.

b. acute lowering of the capnogram values to about zero may indicate a

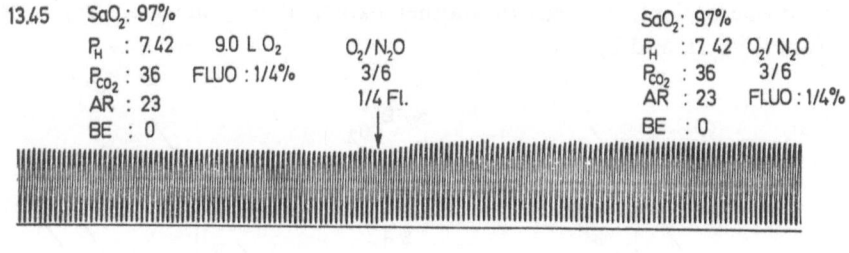

13.45 SaO_2: 97%
      P_H : 7.42   9.0 L O_2 O_2/N_2O
      P_{CO_2} : 36   FLUO : 1/4%   3/6
      AR : 23   1/4 Fl.
      BE : 0

                                               SaO_2: 97%
                                               P_H : 7.42 O_2/N_2O
                                               P_{CO_2} : 36   3/6
                                               AR : 23   FLUO : 1/4%
                                               BE : 0

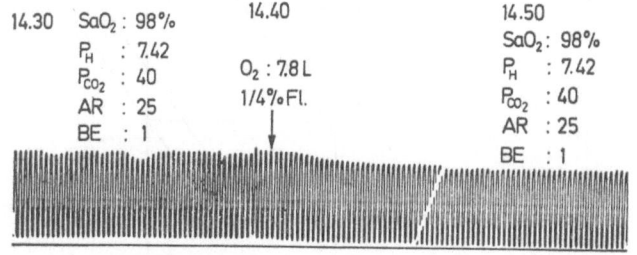

14.30 SaO_2 : 98%   14.40   14.50
      P_H : 7.42 SaO_2: 98%
      P_{CO_2} : 40 O_2 : 7.8 L P_H : 7.42
      AR : 25   1/4% Fl. P_{CO_2} : 40
      BE : 1   AR : 25
                                               BE : 1

Fig. 8. Influence of the F_{IN_2O}.
Changing the F_{IN_2O} from 0% – pure oxygen – to about 66% while keeping total minute ventilation the same, will cause a rise in the inspiratory capnograph readings of about 0.2% and in end-expiratory readings of about 1% due to cross-sensitivity between N_2O and CO_2 in the capnograph.

disconnection in the artificial ventilatory circuit (Fig. 9). Such may easily be converted into an audible alarm to warn the anaesthetist of that event.

c. irregular end-tidal values may indicate insufficient muscle relaxation during the operation (Fig. 10).

d. high or rising end-tidal values after anaesthesia signify insufficient spontaneous ventilation and the need for assisted or controlled ventilation.

SUMMARY

Capnography has proven to be a good measuring/monitoring tool in clinical anaesthesia practice. It may be an excellent trend recorder with regards to carbon dioxide production, its transport to the lungs, and its elimination from the body. It can therefore act as a monitor of metabolism, and of the circulatory and ventilatory systems.

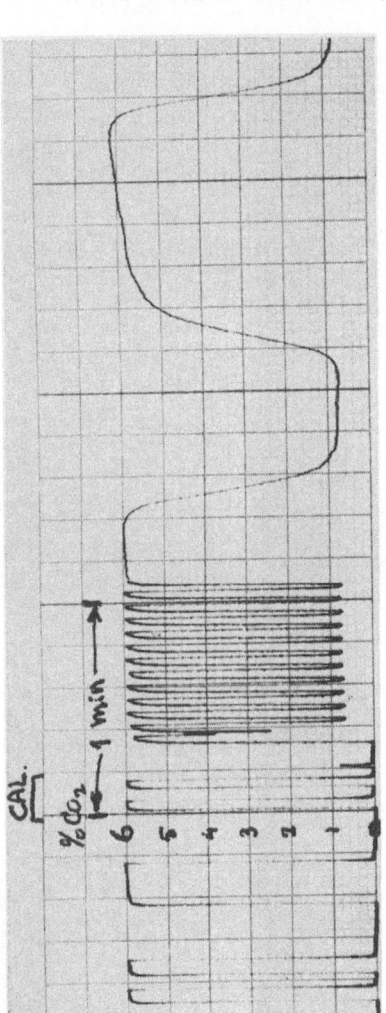

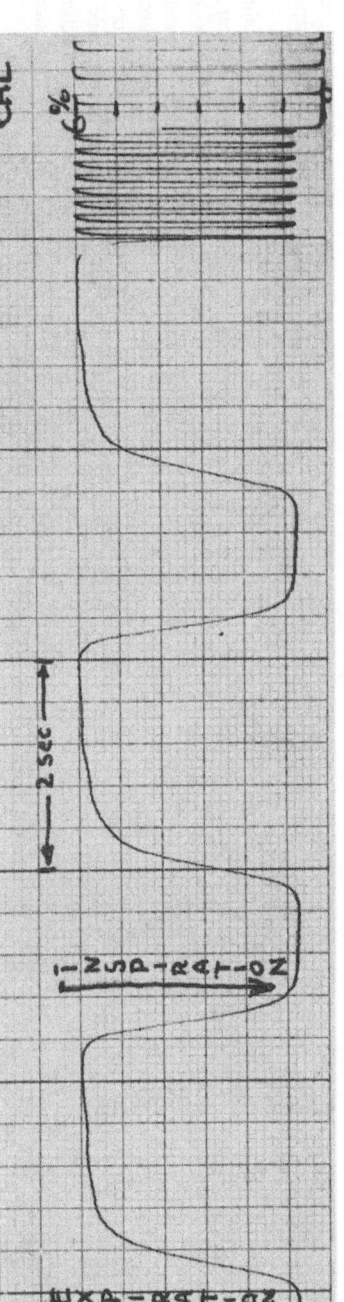

Fig. 1. The normal capnogram of an artificially ventilated patient. 'CAL' = calibration. Below '1 min' the slow recording of expired CO_2 content at a paper speed of 25 mm per min. The lower strip shows three individual breaths, recorded at a writing speed of 750 mm per min, followed by lower speed recording and final calibration. Note that the F_{ICO_2} is not zero, because the sampling point is not directly at the Cobb's piece of the ventilatory circuit, but rather about 10 cm away from it, in the pendulum gas volume between endotracheal tube and ventilatory circuit.

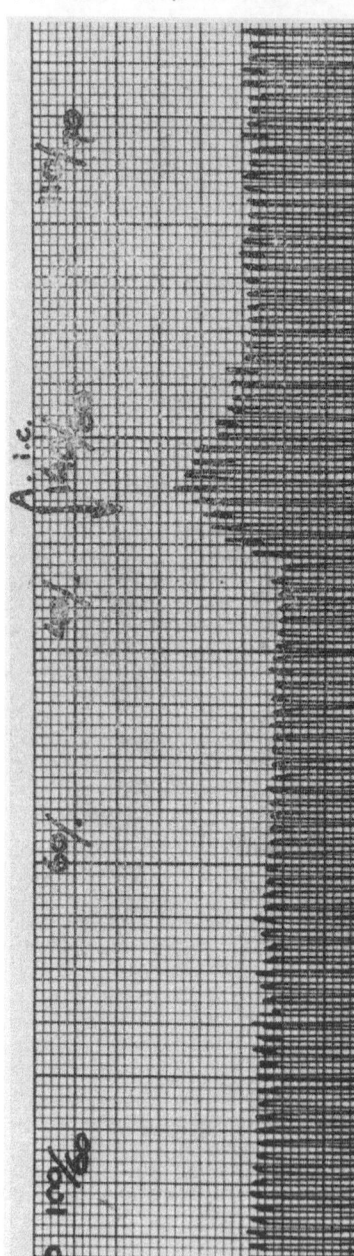

Fig. 2. Behaviour of capnogram during changes in cardiac output and blood pressure.

10 μg of adrenaline were given by intracardiac injection 15 sec before 'A'. The $FE'CO_2$ commenced at 3% and throughout the record follows changes in systemic blood pressure, reflecting pulmonary perfusion (cardiac output).

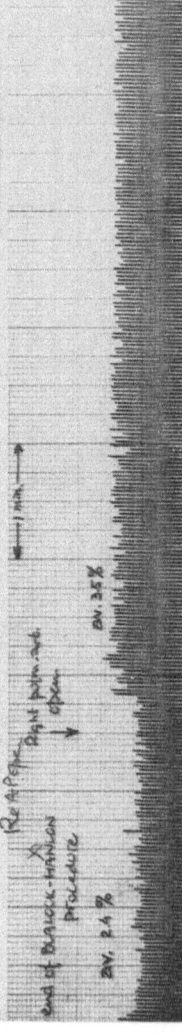

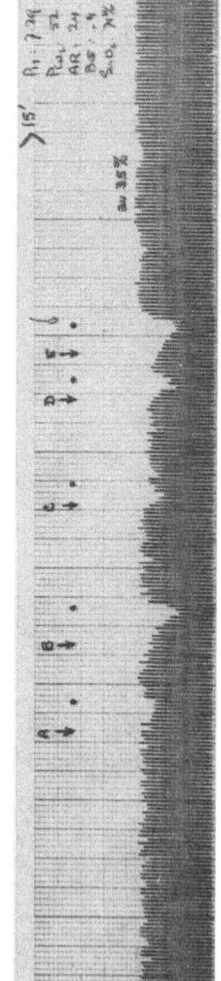

Fig. 3. Capnogram of a patient during a combined Blalock-Hanlon and Damman-Müller operation. After capnographic stabilization following the first procedure (upper strip), attempts to narrow the main pulmonary artery were made at A, B, C, D and E (lower strip).

Acute insufficient pulmonary perfusion is shown at these points, after which – at the dots – the constricting band was released, until – following the last dot – sufficient pulmonary perfusion remained at the same $FECO_2$ level as in the stable period in the upper strip, i.e. as before the constriction.

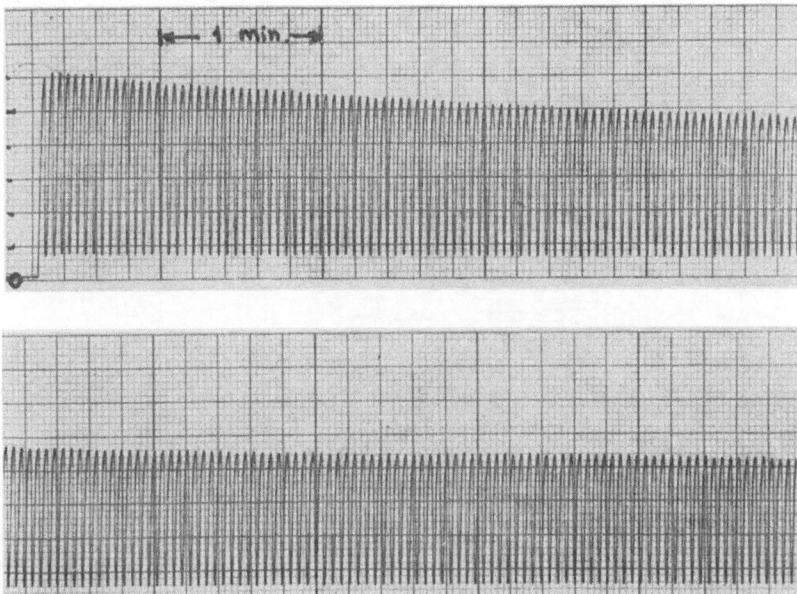

Fig. 4. About thirty seconds after endotracheal intubation a $F_{E'CO_2}$ of 6% was found. After 10 minutes of artificial ventilation this value had diminished to 4.3% and a $PaCO_2$ of 28 Torr was measured. With the aid of a nomogram – Fig. 5 – the ideal $F_{E'CO_2}$ value was determined to be 6%.

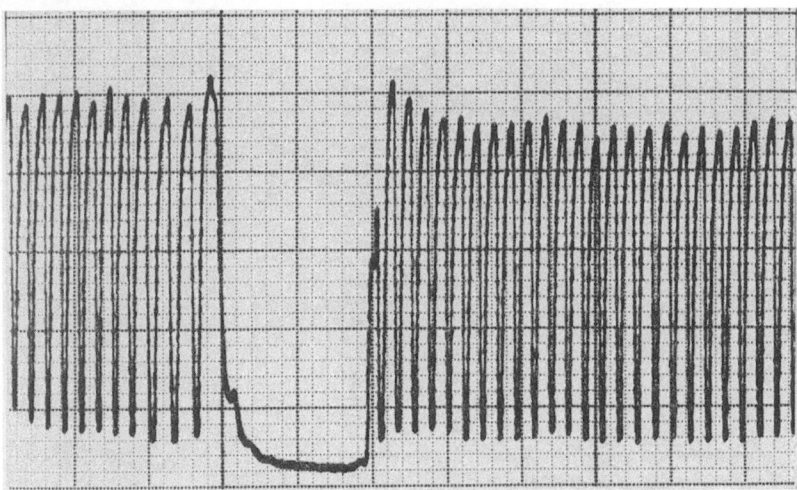

Fig. 9. Disconnection in the ventilatory circuit. This tracing clearly shows the picture of about 20 seconds of zero carbon dioxide removal by artificial ventilation. A gas hose had become disconnected accidentally in the patient's ventilatory circuit. Continuous registrations permits exact knowledge of the duration of such events.

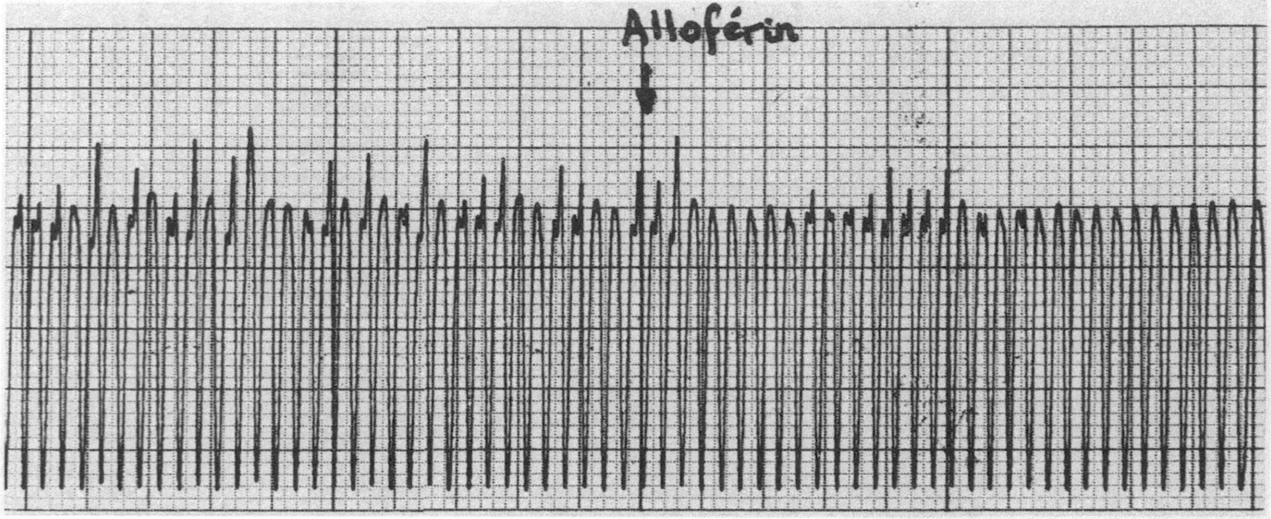

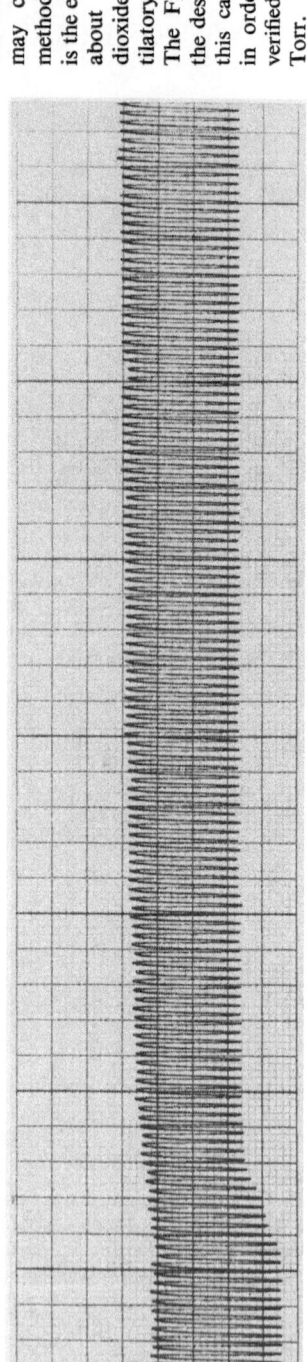

Fig. 10. The influence of insufficient muscle relaxation during anaesthesia. End-expiratory carbon dioxide values are unequal and irregular, due to the patient attempting to breath against the ventilator. About 90 seconds after an intravenous dose of alcuronium (Alloférin®) the end-tidal values for carbon dioxide again become equal, regular and stable.

Fig. 6. In order to increase the $F_{E'CO_2}$ to the desired level one may choose several methods. Shown here is the effect of adding about 1% carbon dioxide in the ventilatory gas mixture. The $F_{E'CO_2}$ rises to the desired value – in this case to 5.0% – in order to attain a verified $PaCO_2$ of 40 Torr.

CAPNOGRAPHY 87

Under circumstances of constant carbon dioxide production and normal circulatory conditions there is a relationship between the capnometric values and the $PaCO_2$. If any deviation from normal conditions is to be expected – and such may often well be the case during anaesthesia and surgery –, it would seem wise to 'calibrate' the capnograph with at least one initial $PaCO_2$ value.

Continuous capnography may be used as a monitor of technical equipment failure, such as leaks in or disconnection of ventilatory gas hoses.

Furthermore the capnograph, when used at higher writing speeds may be used to study peculiarities of individual breaths: among others, the necessity for an additional dose of relaxant may be readily detected.

REFERENCES

1. Digby Leigh, M., Jenkins, L. C., Bilton, M. K. & Lewis, J. B., Continuous alveolar carbon dioxide analysis as a monitor of pulmonary blood flow. *Anesthesiology* 18, 878 (1957).
2. Digby Leigh, M., Jones, J. C. & Motley H. L., The expired carbon dioxide as a continuous guide of the pulmonary and circulatory systems during anaesthesia and surgery. *J. Thorac. Cardiovasc. Surg.* 41, 597 (1961).
3. Burton, G. W., The value of carbon dioxide monitoring during anaesthesia. *Anaesthesia* 21, 173 (1966).
4. Smalhout, B., *Capnography*. Its importance in diagnosis, operation, and aftertreatment of neurosurgical patients. Thesis Utrecht 1967. A. Oosthoek's uitgeversmaatschappij N.V. Utrecht.
5. Luft, K., Über eine neue Methode der registrierenden Gasanalyse mit Hilfe der Absorbtion ultraroter Strahlen ohne spektrale Zerlegung. *Ztschr. Techn. Phys.* 24, 97 (1943).
6. Janssen, P. J., The value of capnography in the Dammann–Müller operation. *Der Anaesthesist* 21, 37 (1972).
7. Janssen, P. J., A pitfall in capnographic monitoring during anaesthesia. *Anaesthesist* 21, 29 (1972).
8. Hill, D. W. & Powell, T., Cross-sensitivity effects in nondispersive infra-red gas analysers using condenser microphone detectors. *J. Sci. Instrum.* 44, 189 (1967).

PNEUMOTACHOGRAPHY

G. ROLLY AND L. RENDERS–VERSICHELEN

Pneumotachography is a method for measuring gas flow during respiration. More than 45 years ago Fleisch (1) first described the pneumotachograph. It is the aim of this chapter to discuss this technique in some detail and to focus on both the clinical applications and possible errors in the technique.

TYPES OF PNEUMOTACHOGRAPHS

A pneumotachograph is essentially a small resistance to gas flow, which is placed in series with the gas flow to be measured. The physical principle behind the instrument is the law of Poisseuille, which states that under conditions of laminar flow, the flow of a gas is directly proportional to the driving pressure gradient. The design of the pneumotachograph is such that the flow through it is laminar and the pressure drop appearing accross the head, is linearly related to the gas velocity, up to a specific maximum flow. A sensitive manometer is connected across the head and can be calibrated in terms of gas velocity or flow rate. The fact that the resistance to flow of the head is small and usually of the order of a few mm H_2O means that it can be inserted into a breathing circuit with minimal interruption to the respiration of the patient.

Two types of pneumotachographs are used for clinical application. One pneumotachograph head is that of Fry, and consists of a sheet of fine-mesh wire gauze, inserted in a tube. On each side of the mesh, connections are provided to the two sides of a sensitive differential pressure manometer. The pneumotachograph is electrically heated to prevent condensation of expired water vapour.

The most popular pneumotachograph head ,however, is that of Fleisch which consists of a large number of small, parallel metal tubes, inserted in a greater tube. It is made by rolling a sheet of thin corrugated metal with a plane strip of metal. It is also heated to prevent condensation of water vapour during exhalation. The two endings are again connected to a differential pressure manometer. Several different sizes of the Fleisch head are available (N° 00 - 4).

These range in volume from 1.7 ml to 200 ml, and cover a range of flows from a few liters per minute to 1,000 liters per minute. In each case the pressure drop developed from the maximum flow rate is of the order of 7 mm H_2O.

With a small size pneumotachograph the linearity of response is limited to slow flows. With an increasing size, a large dead space is added to the patients airways if both the inspired and expired gases pass through it.

CALIBRATION OF THE DEVICE

The calibration of the pneumatachograph head in terms of flow rate, is accomplished by passing known gas flows through it.

The flows can be produced by a compressor and measured by a rotameter type flowmeter. If the output of the pressure manometer can be connected to a fast writing recorder then another method of calibration is possible, using a sine wave pump (Fig. 1). This was originally described by Cooper (2) and Hill, Hook and Bell (3), and later improved by Herzog and Norlander (4, 5). A small piston pump is used, with known characteristics of velocity, capacity, etc. Accordingly the peak gas flow is exactly known.

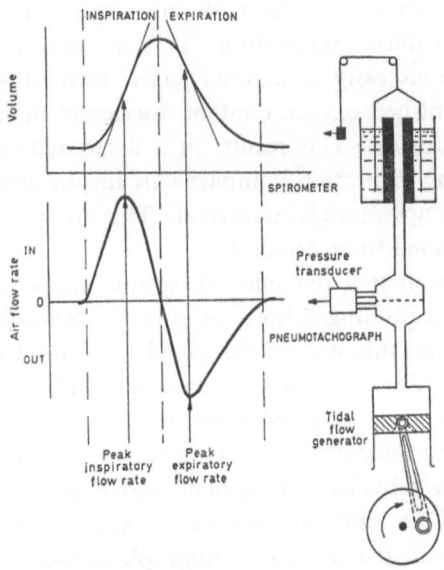

Fig. 1. Calibration of the pneumotachograph.
(From J. F. Nunn, Applied respiratory physiology, Butterworths, London 1969).

The next point to take into consideration is that actual measurements under clinical conditions are often with *other* gas mixtures, than those used for calibration. Errors can be made due to the differences in molecular weight and hence in viscosity, of air, oxygen, and nitrous oxide (Table 1).

Table 1. Viscosity of some gases and possible error.

Gas	Viscosity at + 20 °C in centipoises	Error of volume in % on calibration with air
Air	0.0183	0
Oxygen	0.0202	+ 9.4
Nitrogen	0.0175	− 4.6
Carbon dioxide	0.0148	−23.6
Nitrous oxide	0.0146	−25.3

If calibration is undertaken with air alone and measurements are performed with other gases, large errors are introduced. This error will be of + 9% if oxygen is used after calibration with air, but during anaesthesia with 70% nitrous oxide, the volume can be underestimated by 20%. Calibration should therefore always be made with the inspired mixture. Changes in viscosity also occur during respiration. This is due to the differences in gas composition. The viscosity of expired gas is lower than that of inspired gas owing to diminished oxygen content, increased humidity, and the presence of carbon dioxide. This results in a decreased reading of the same volume flow during expiration compared to inspiration, if only gas composition and not temperature is concerned. This error is, however, relatively small and is calculated to be about 2%.

Another point is that a pneumotachograph needs frequent calibration when used during a prolonged time. A suitable device has been developed for that purpose and this will be described in some detail. The pneumotachocalibrator (4,5) enables an instantaneous calibration of the pneumotachograph, before each series of measurements, by using the actual gas mixture breathed by the patient (6). This calibration device consists mainly of two parts: a switchvalve arrangment and a small piston pump. The pneumotachograph is built into the switch-valve and can be set in two positions: either with the pneumotachograph in the respiratory circuit of the patient or with the pneumotachograph in the calibrating circuit. An electrically driven small piston pump with exactly known characteristics is used to calibrate the pneumotachograph, by introducing a known gas at a known flow rate at regular intervals. The exhaled respiratory gases of the patient can be used for calibration.

In addition, a pressure of known intensity is provided intermittently for calibrating the pressure transducer. The whole process of calibration before each measurement, can be made in about 10 seconds. The heating of the pneumotachograph to avoid condensation and hence turbulent flow, increases the temperature of the gases passingt hrough it, which must be taken into consideration. On the other hand the pneumotachograph head cannot be heated very strongly because of possible danger to the patient.

It has been shown that the output increases by 1% for each degree temperature rise when raising the temperature from ambient to 37 °C, and the output decreases by 1.2% when saturating dry air, at the same temperature (7). Calibration must be arranged in such a way that the conditions of the gases are as similar as possible to the conditions during the measurements.

INSERTION IN THE BREATHING CIRCUIT

The place of the pneumotachograph in the breathing circuit needs consideration for several reasons. The respiratory gases differ in their physical properties during the different phases of the breathing cycle. In normal spontaneous respiration the inspired gas is of ambient temperature and humidity. During expiration, the gas is at body temperature and saturated with water vapour. If, however, the pneumotachograph is placed in such a way that only the inspired or expired gas is passing through the pneumotachograph, the situation is considerably simplified.

This is easy to arrange during spontaneous respiration, but difficult during controlled ventilation. Compression of the respiratory gases takes place during the inspiratory period within the ventilator and the tubing.

If the pneumotachograph is placed either at the inflow or at the outflow tube, large errors may be induced during controlled ventilation. When both the inspired and expired gases pass through the pneumotachograph, the expired volume is in fact different from the inspired one, and this will need an automatic zero reset for obtaining the volume curves (see later).

The use of a pneumotachograph is in general simple with spontaneously breathing patients. But during intermittent positive pressure ventilation, care must be taken to use thick walled tubing between the pneumotachographic head and the manometer. During controlled ventilation, with the high pressure generated, the Fleisch pneumotachograph is suitable.

USE OF PNEUMOTACHOGRAPH

The primary use of the pneumotachograph is to provide measurements and recordings of *actual and peak gas flow rates*; this is a very useful information during studies of breathing patterns and testing of ventilators. Clinically, the anaesthetist is more interested in the *tidal volume* of the patient and hence minute volume. This can easily be done by electrically integrating, the output from the pneumotachograph transducer, with respect to time. The volume curve shows an upward curve corresponding to inspiration, the peak height giving the tidal inspired volume, and a downward curve corresponding to expiration.

Taking into account the difficulties already mentioned, both inspiratory and expiratory volumes are equal if the respiratory quotient is 1, but normally they are not as the respiratory quotient is mostly around 0.85 during anaesthesia.

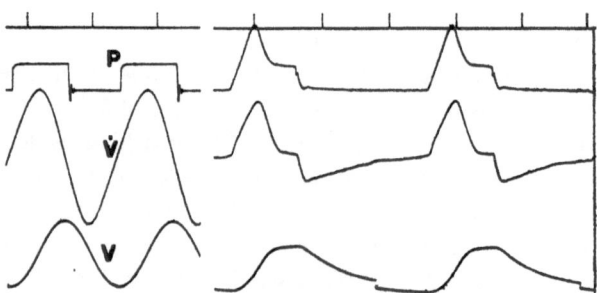

Fig. 2. Automatic zero reset of volume curve; from top to bottom: pressure, flow, volume.

In order to prevent drifting of the baseline, an automatic reset mechanism is usually built in (Fig. 2). An automatic reset to the zero line is also possible after both inspiration and expiration. This allows a separate graphic recording of both inspiratory and expiratory volumes (Fig. 3). To record the *minute volume*, the output signal from the pneumotachograph pressure transducer is passed through a halfwave rectifier and in this case the record consists of a staircase-like tracing, each step being a tidal volume (Fig. 4).

The integrator can be reset after a preset volume or a preset time.

For lung function studies various auxiliary electronic circuits can be provided; for example a circuit to store the peak value of inspiratory or expiratory flow rate. This can be displayed in numerical values. A volume recording can also be made. The value of the total volume after 1 sec. (FEV₁). Figure 3 shows a separate recording of the flow in addition to the original and the quotient therefrom, as well as those for calculation of the inspiratory expiratory ratio (Fig. 3).

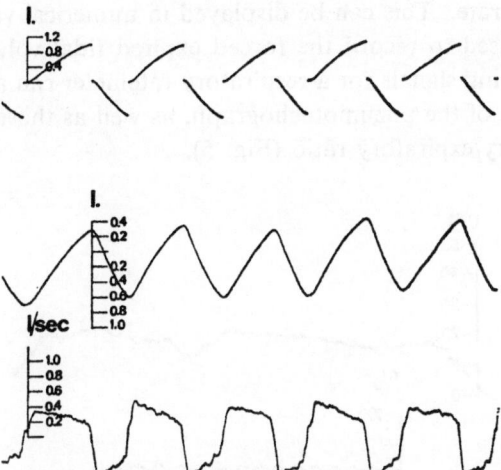

Fig. 3. Separate recording of inspiratory and expiratory volumes (upper trace); normal volume recording (middle trace); flow recording (lower trace). (By courtesy of Godart-Statham – Holland).

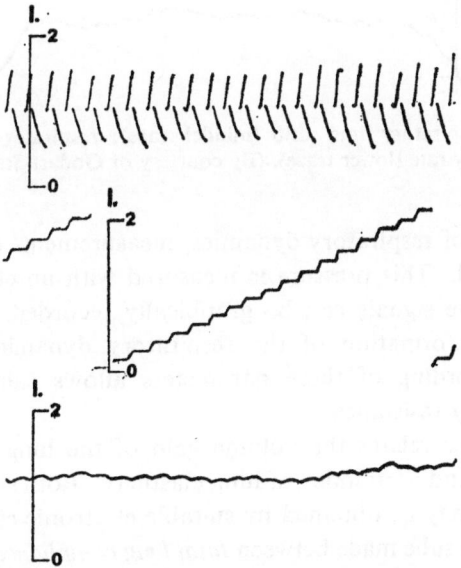

Fig. 4. Staircase integration of inspiratory volume (middle trace); separate recording of inspiratory and expiratory volumes (upper trace); mean respiratory flow rate (lower trace). (By courtesy of Godart-Statham – Holland).

expiratory flow rate. This can be displayed in numerical values. A timing circuit can be used to record the forced expired tidal volume after 1 sec. 'FEV$_1$'. Triggering signals for a respiratory ratemeter can also be obtained from the output of the pneumotachograph, as well as those for calculation of the inspiratory/expiratory ratio (Fig. 5).

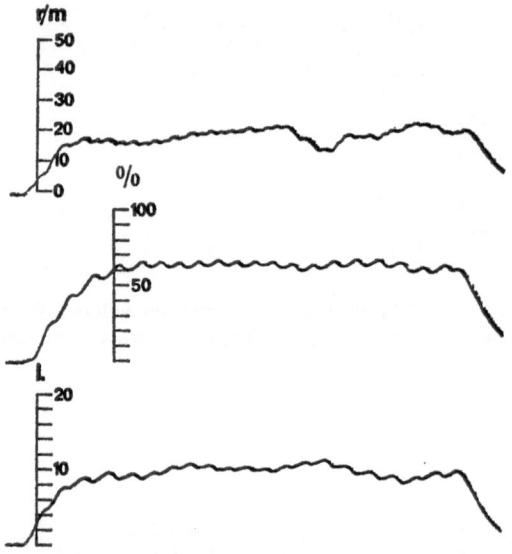

Fig. 5. Inspiratory/expiratory time ratio (middel trace); respiratory rate (upper trace); mean respiratory flow rate (lower trace). (By courtesy of Godart-Statham – Holland).

For most studies of respiratory dynamics, measurements of pressure in the airways are added. This pressure is measured with an electronic pressure transducer and the signals can be graphically recorded. This gives even more complete information of the respiratory dynamics (Fig. 6). The simultaneous recording of these parameters allows calculation of compliance and airway resistance.

Lung compliance relates the volume gain of the lung for each unit of pressure increase and is an index of lung elasticity. Both static and dynamic lung compliance may be obtained by suitable electronic circuitory.

A distinction must be made between *total lung compliance, lung compliance* and *chest wall compliance*, relating the change in lung volume respectively to the change in alveolar/ambient pressure gradient, alveolar/intrathoracic pressure gradient and ambient/intrathoracic pressure gradient.

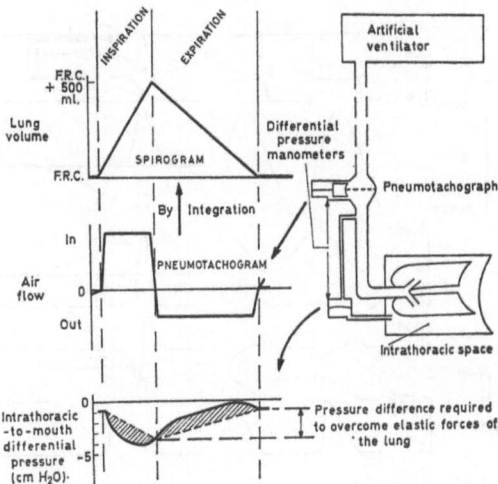

Fig. 6. Simultaneous recording of flow, volume and pressure. (From J. F. Nunn, Applied respiratory physiology, Butterworths, London 1969).

Airway resistance is the resistance against flow. It is the pressure difference along the airways divided by the gas flow. This value is commonly quoted in the literature for a gasflow of 0.5 l/sec. Automatic calculation of airway resistance is not easy and very few devices give a reliable value. It is calculated during spontaneous respiration, using whole body plethysmography. A more time consuming method consists of calculating resistance using the tracings of pneumotachography. During controlled respiration the measured pressure is due partly to the volume insufflated for expanding the lungs (the so-called compliance pressure) and partly to resistance against insufflation (the resistance pressure) (Table 2). By calculating the instantaneous pressure relative to the momentary insufflated volume, the pressure relative to resistance can be deduced and accordingly the airway resistance can be computed (Fig. 7).

Table 2. Derivation of total pressure, for calculation of resistance.

$$P = P \text{ compl.} + P \text{ resist.}$$

$$P = \frac{V}{C_{TL}} + R_{TL} \cdot V$$

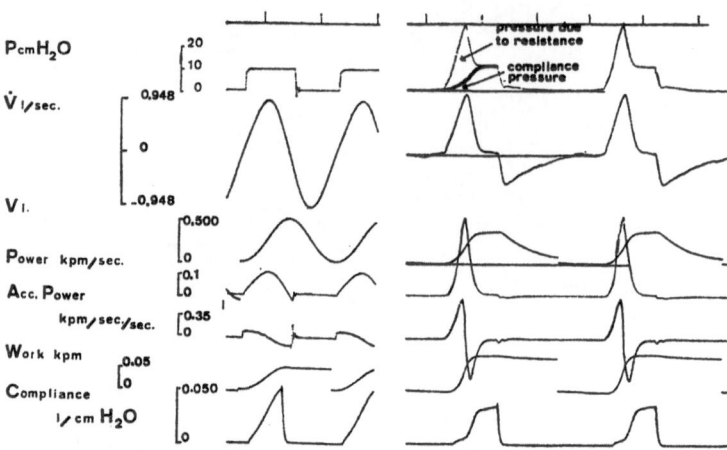

Fig. 7. Derivation of airway resistance.

From the three fundamental values of flow, volume and pressure, other values can be calculated electronically.

Actual respiratory power is the product of pressure and flow (8) (Table 3). Dividing the actual respiratory power by time provides the acceleration of respiratory power (dPower/dt). *Respiratory work* is the integration of respiratory power during one inspiratory cycle.

Table 3. Units.

— Pressure (P)	cm H_2O
— Flow ($\dot{V}$)	l/sec
— Volume (V)	l
— Power ($= k. \triangle p. \Lambda$)	kpm/sec*
(k is a constant $= 0.01$)	
— Acceleration of Power (dPower/$_{dt}$)	kpm/sec/sec
— Work (W)	kpm
— Compliance ($\dfrac{V}{p}$)	l/cm H_2O
— Resistance ($\dfrac{p}{\dot{V}}$)	cm H_2O/l/sec
* (kpm = kilopound meter)	

CLINICAL APPLICATIONS

Using pneumotachography, it is possible to measure the different respiratory parameters in the spontaneously breathing patient, as well as in the patient during controlled respiration. This can be done in short-duration anaesthesia, or during prolonged ventilatory treatment. The evolution of certain respiratory parameters with time, is very important. Lung compliance has been studied during short-duration ventilation in this way. It was shown that there were no changes with time during controlled ventilation, at least with the Engström respirator (9).

Rapidly changing respiratory parameters during cardiopulmonary by-pass have also been studied (10). The influence of acute administration of pharmacological drugs can also be tested easily (11).

The method can be applied, without difficulty, to the testing of ventilators under experimental conditons (10, 12, 13). Two artificial lungs have been built for this purpose and consist of two large glass bottles, partly filled with water. The water filling is intended to maintain the adiabatic compression. The compliance is similar to that normally found during anaesthesia, and by eliminating one bottle a 50% reduction of compliance can be simulated. The conducting tubing has a normal resistance but additional resistances can be incorporated to simulate increased airway resistance.

As an illustration of this technique, the testing of the Servoventilator can be analysed. When using an increasing flow pattern and a driving pressure

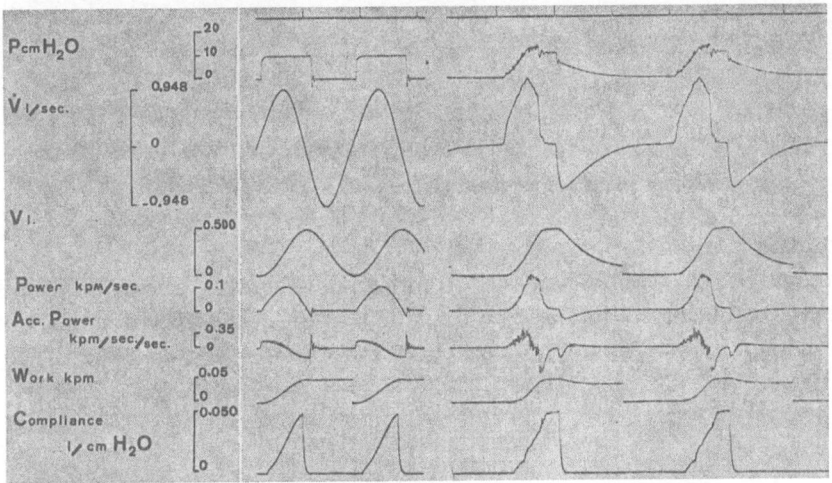

Fig. 8. Servoventilator: increasing flow pattern.

of 80 cm H_2O with this ventilator, a simultaneous increase and peak value of the pressure and flow curves are noticed (14), furthermore, the respiratory power increases accordingly, with a maximum value coinciding with the other peak (Fig. 8). The time derivation of respiratory power $(dPower/_{dt})$ is positive during the greatest part of the insufflation period and becomes negative only just before the peak value of power. At the end of inspiration, a static pressure plateau is present. These tracings closely resemble those previously described for the Engström respirator (6). The constant flow pattern gives a nearly square flow wave with a linear increase in pressure, followed by a pressure plateau, during the no flow period (Fig. 9).
The peak of respiratory power is occurring at the end of the insufflation period. The time derivate, however, is most positive at the early beginning of the inspiratory period.

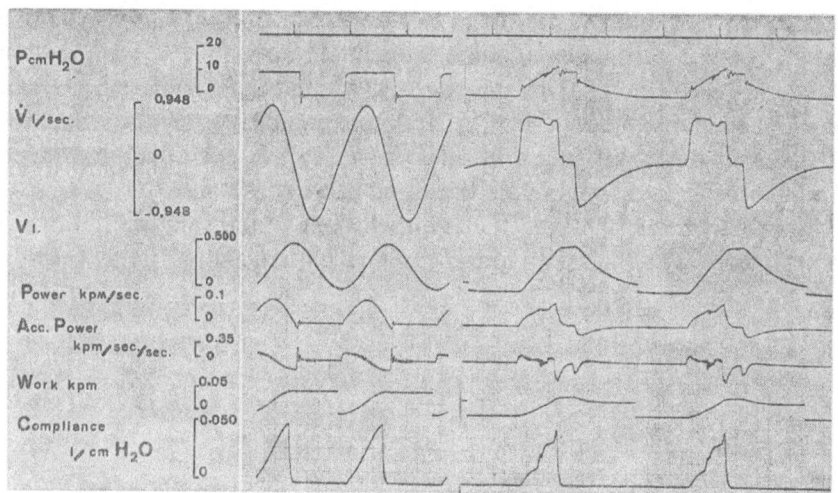

Fig. 9. Servoventilator: constant flow pattern.

CONCLUSION

This survey of the possibilities of pneumotachography shows that this method is of clinical importance for studying the respiratory dynamics of the patient as well as its use for research purposes.

REFERENCES

1. Fleisch, A., Der Pneumotachograph: die Apparatur zur Geschwindigkeitsregistrierung der Atemluft. *Pflügers Arch. Ges. Physiol.*, 209, 713 (1925).
2. Cooper, E. A., Behaviour of respiratory apparatus. *Medical Research Memorandum*, 2, II, London, National Coal Board, 1961.
3. Hill, D. W., Hook, J. R. & Bell, E. G., Servo-operated respiratory waveform simulator. *J. Scient. Instrum.*, 38, 100 (1961).
4. Herzog, P. & Norlander, O. P., Praecisions-Instrument für die Eichung von Pneumotachographen. *Anaesthesist*, 15, 168-169 (1966).
5. Herzog, P. & Norlander, O. P., A precision method for the dynamic volume-flow calibration during pneumotachography. *Acta Anaesth. Scand.*, suppl. XXIV, 119-126 (1966).
6. Rolly, G. & Malcolm–Thomas, B., Modern technique of measuring pulmonary ventilation. First experience. *Acta Anaesth. Belg.*, 24, 48-57 (1973).
7. Hobbes, A. F. T., A comparison of methods of calibrating the pneumotachograph. *Brit. J. Anaesth.*, 39, 899 (1967).
8. Engström, C. G. & Norlander, O. P., A new method for analysis of respiratory work by measurements of the actual power as a function of gas flow, pressure and time. *Acta Anaesth. Scand.*, 6, 49-55 (1962).
9. Norlander, O. P., Herzog, P., Norden, I., Hossli, G., Schaer, H. & Gattiker, R., Compliance and airway resistance during anesthesia with controlled ventilation. *Acta Anaesth. Scand.*, 12, 135-152 (1968).
10. Baum, M., Bednarik, M., Benzer, H., Domanig, E., Haider, W., Lepier, W., Niessner, G., Rieder, W. & Tölle, W., Veränderungen der Atemmechanik während Operationen am offenen Herzen (Zusammenhänge zwischen Herz-Kreislauffunktion und Atemmechanik). *III. Congressus Anaesthesiologicus Europaeus*, Praga, 749, 1970.
11. Meloche, R., Norlander, O., Norden, I. & Herzog, P., Effects of carbon dioxide and halothane on compliance and pulmonary resistance during cardio-pulmonary bypass. *Scand. J. Thor. Cardiov. Surg.*, 3, 69-78 (1969).
12. Norlander, O. P., Functional analysis of force and power of mechanical ventilators. *Acta Anaesth. Scand.*, 8, 57-77 (1964).
13. Herzog, P. & Norlander, O. P., Distribution of alveolar volumes with different types of positive pressure gasflow patterns. *Opuscula Medica*, 1, 3-18 (1968).
14. Rolly, G. & Malcolm–Thomas, B., Functional evaluation of the servoventilator. Presented at the German Congress of Anaesthesiology, Hamburg 1972; to be published in Der Anaesthesist.

GAS CHROMATOGRAPHY AND THE ANALYSIS OF VOLATILE ANAESTHETIC AGENTS IN RESPIRATORY GASES AND IN BLOOD

A. G. L. BURM, H. H. BENEKEN KOLMER AND C. A. CRAMERS

During anaesthesia and recovery, the condition of the patient is determined to a large extent by the type and the dose of the anaesthetic agent administered. Therefore it is essential that anaesthetists know at all times how much aneasthetic is being administered to the patient.

In most cases the dose is estimated from the setting of the vaporiser. However, differences may exist between the dial setting of the vaporiser and the actual concentration in the inspiratory gas mixture, see Fig. 1. Many vaporisers show hysteresis and ,in addition, the concentration is often dependent on the total gas flow. From these facts it can be concluded that an analysis of anaesthetics in inspiratory gas mixtures might be desirable.

The concentrations in alveoli and in blood are even more important,

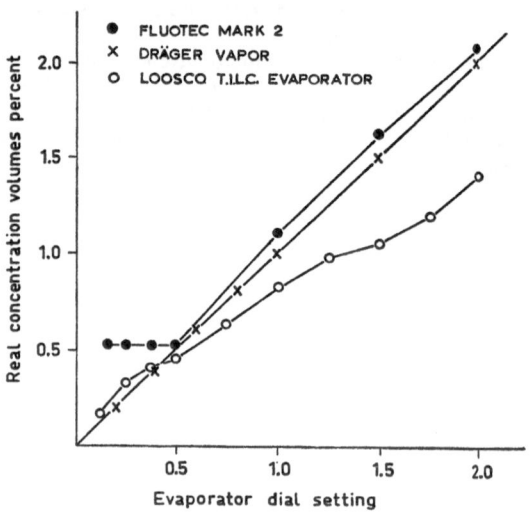

Fig. 1. Actual concentration versus dial setting.

since they are probably correlated to the anaesthetic action. Measurement of these concentrations, together with a thorough knowledge of the pharmacokinetics of anaesthetic agents, can contribute to improved patient care.

This article describes some methods for gas chromatographic analysis of volatile anaesthetic agents in respiratory gases and in blood which are used in an investigation of the pharmacokinetics of halothane (1-5). A short description of the principles of gas chromatography is given first.

BASIC CONCEPTS OF GAS CHROMATOGRAPHY

Gas chromatography is a collective name for a group of analytical separation methods used for the analysis of volatile substances in the gas phase (6-7). They all have in common that the substances to be analysed are distributed between two phases. One of these phases is stationary, the other is mobile. The latter phase is gas flowing past the former. The stationary phase may be a solid adsorbent (Gas Solid Chromatography, GSC) or it may be a liquid made stationary by distributing it over an inert support (Gas Liquid Chromatography, GLC). The stationary phase is packed in a glass or metal column; common dimensions are 2 meters long and 1/8 inch inner diameter.

A quantity describing the distribution of a solute between the two phases is the partition coefficient, K, defined by:

$$K = \frac{C_s}{C_m} \qquad [1]$$

where

C_s, concentration solute in stationary phase

C_m, concentration solute in mobile phase

The mobile phase is a gas that is not retained by the stationary phase, e.g. helium or nitrogen. Its role is to carry the sample molecules through the chromatographic column, hence the name carrier gas.

A schematic diagram of a gas chromatograph is presented in Fig. 2. The sample is usually introduced by means of a microsyringe into the carrier gas stream at the inlet of the column (injection port). For the introduction of gaseous samples special sample valves have been developed. During transport through the column the individual sample components are retarded, each according to its affinity for the stationary phase. The partition coefficient, and hence the residence time of the sample components, is highly influenced by the column temperature. Therefore the column is placed in a precisely controlled oven. At the column outlet there is a device, the detector, which indicates the presence of the compounds emerging at differ-

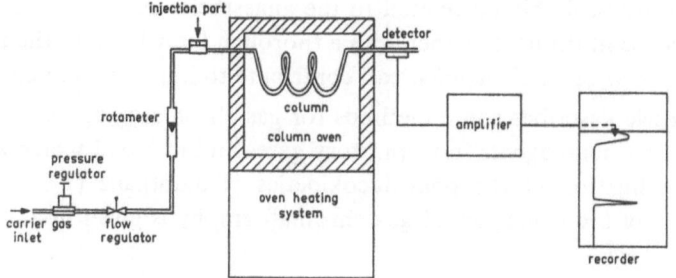

Fig. 2. Scheme of a gas chromatograph.

ent times in the carrier gas. The signal of the detector plotted as a function of time is called a chromatogram, Fig. 3. The time which elapses between the emergence of the peak maximum and the injection of the sample is called the retention time. Retention times, or derivatives thereof, are used in qualitative analysis. The area of a peak, or in some cases the peak height, is proportional to the quantity of the component.

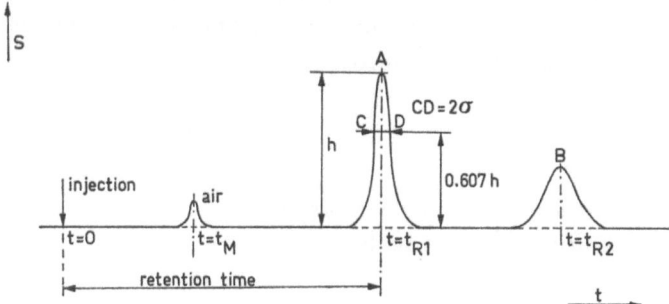

Fig. 3. Chromatogram with definition of common terms.

The actual separation of two components is affected by the difference in their retention times and by the peak broadening which is due to several diffusion phenomena. A measure of the 'goodness' of a column with respect to peak broadening is the so-called plate number n. A larger plate number (smaller peak width) means better separation power.

RETENTION TIME

The residence time of the peak maximum in the column, the retention time t_R (sec) in the case of GLC, is given by:

$$t_R = \frac{L}{\bar{u}}\left(1 + K\frac{V_L}{V_G}\right) = t_M\left(1 + K\frac{V_L}{V_G}\right) \qquad [2]$$

where

t_R,	retention time (measured from start)
L,	length of the column (cm)
$\bar{u}$,	average velocity of the mobile phase (cm/sec)
K,	partition coefficient
$L/\bar{u} = t_M$,	gas holdup time, the retention time of an unretained component (e.g. air or the carrier gas itself)
V_L,	volume of stationary phase in the column (cm³)
V_G,	volume of mobile phase in the column (cm³)

The phase ratio V_L/V_G in packed columns is on the order of 0,05 - 0,1. It may be concluded that substances with different K values have different retention times in a column. K is dependent on the vapour pressure of the components at the column temperature as well as the nature of the components and the stationary phase. Careful selection of the stationary phase allows separation of compounds with exactly the same boiling points.

PEAK BROADENING

A narrow and concentrated zone of a solute, such as is introduced at the column inlet, broadens in time to a wider band (compare peak A and B in Fig. 3). A quantity describing this phenomenon is the plate number, n, of the column given by:

$$n = \frac{t_R^2}{\sigma^2} \qquad [3]$$

where

n, number of plates

σ^2, variance (in time square units) of the eluted peak.

The standard deviation σ can be derived from the chromatogram as follows (for symmetrical gaussian peaks, see fig. 3):

$$\sigma = \frac{CD}{2}; \qquad CD, \text{ width at 0.607 height} \qquad [4]$$

The plate number is a function of the linear velocity $\bar{u}$ of the carrier gas and a number of experimental parameters.

RESOLUTION

The degree of separation of two components leaving the column shortly after one another can be expressed by the resolution R. This quantity is defined by, see Fig. 4:

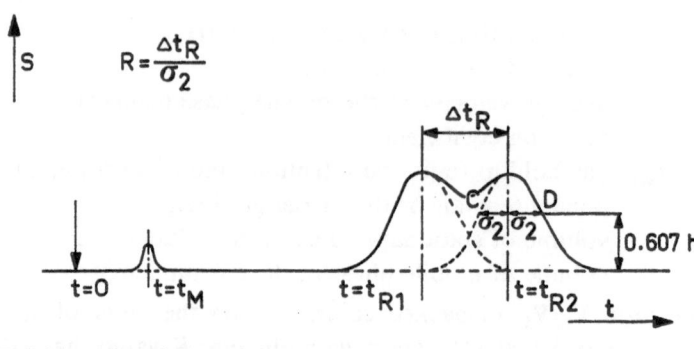

Fig. 4. Definition of resolution.

$$R = \frac{t_{R2} - t_{R1}}{\sigma_2} \qquad [5]$$

With [3] this becomes:

$$R = \frac{t_{R2} - t_{R1}}{t_{R2}} \sqrt{n} = (1 - \frac{t_{R1}}{t_{R2}}) \sqrt{n} \qquad [6]$$

n, the plate number is proportional to the length of the column. The separation is almost complete if R = 6 and just acceptable if R = 4.

A number of stationary phases are available in selected separation problems to make $t_{R2} - t_{R1}$ as large as possible. However, for a very complex sample containing substances of different chemical classes it is difficult to maximize Δt_R for all components. The only way to effect a separation then is to use high resolution columns. Columns with over a million theoretical plates have been described.

QUALITATIVE ANALYSIS

Qualitative analysis in GLC is carried out by comparing retention times or derivatives thereof with values obtained from known samples. This implies that the column temperature must be known with great precision (say 0.2 °C) and must be constant throughout its length.

A column temperature increase of say 30 °C roughly decreases K (and hence also t_R) by a factor of 3. This has been put to use in the so-called programmed temperature technique. During the analysis the column temperature is increased linearly at a specific rate. In this way products with a wide boiling range may be analysed in one run. High boiling point trace components are concentrated in this way and can be detected better.

QUANTITATIVE ANALYSIS

As said before the peak area (or the peak height) is proportional to the sample concentration. In general, resolution decreases with increasing sample size. The smallest possible sample size, however, is determined by the detection system selected. Sample sizes in gas chromatography range from 10^{-12} to 10^{-2} grams.

CHROMATOGRAPHY DETECTORS

Since the introduction of gas chromatography several detectors have been developed, each with its own applications (8). The choice of the right detector is mainly determined by the nature and the concentrations of the components in the samples to be analysed. For the detection of respiratory gases and anaesthetic agents a choice can be made from the following detectors:

a) The *katharometer*, which is based on the difference in thermal conductivity between the carrier gas and the components. The sensitivity of this detector is dependent on the carrier gas used. If the quantities of the substances in the samples are small a carrier gas of high thermal conductivity, e.g. helium, should be used.

The katharometer is able to detect all components, but it has a low sensitivity in comparison with the other detectors described here. In anaesthesiology it is used for the detection of O_2, N_2, CO_2 and N_2O in samples of respiratory gases or blood. In some cases it is also used for the detection of organic anaesthetic agents.

b) The *ultrasonic detector*, which is based on the fact that the velocity of sound in a gas mixture is dependent on the composition of the mixture. This detector has a higher sensitivity than the katharometer, but expensive equipment is necessary.

The ultrasonic detector is used for the detection of O_2, N_2, CO_2 and N_2O from blood samples (2). It is very appropriate for measurement during recovery, when the concentration of N_2O decreases quickly.

c) The *flame ionization detector*, which is based on the fact that organic compounds are partially ionized when they are burnt in a hydrogen-air flame.

This very sensitive detector is used for the detection of organic anaesthetic agents. It cannot be used for the detection of inorganic gases as the latter are not ionized.

d) The *electron capture detector*. In this ionization detector with a radio-active source, use is made of the fact that some compounds can absorb electrons from a 'standing current'. The electron capture detector has a very high sensitivity and selectivity, which can be profitable. Its use is somewhat restricted because the response of the detector is only proportional to the quantity of the substances at low concentrations. Therefore it is used only for the detection of very small amounts of halogenated hydrocarbons, e.g. halogenated anaesthetic agents in highly diluted solutions of heptane or benzene, obtained by extraction of blood samples.

Another application of the electron capture detector is the measurement of traces of halogenated anaesthetics in the air of operating theatres or recovery rooms.

ANALYSIS OF ORGANIC ANAESTHETIC AGENTS IN RESPIRATORY GASES

The concentration of organic anaesthetic agents in respiratory gases can be determined by injecting a small sample into the gas chromatograph. Fig. 5 shows the chromatogram obtained after injection of a sample of air containing some common anaesthetics and acetone. The concentration of the components varied from 0.1 to 0.7 volume percent. Acetone was included in the analysis because small quantities may be present in expiratory gases in pathological cases.

The analysis was carried out with a Perkin Elmer 900 gas chromatograph. Separation took place in a 20 cm stainless steel column (inner diameter 3/32 inch), packed with Porasil S + Carbowax 400 (80 - 100 mesh). For the detection of the components a flame ionization detector was used.

Further data are:

— carrier gas   : nitrogen, flow 55 ml/min
— injection port temperature : 100 °C
— column temperature   : 60 °C
— detector temperature   : 150 °C
— injection   : 200 µl gas

The concentrations of anaesthetic agents in samples of unknown composition are derived from measurement of the peak height. In a series of 25 injections

retention times

diethyl ether	18.2"
acetone	32.4ˢ
trilene	1'10.2"
halothane	1'53.2"

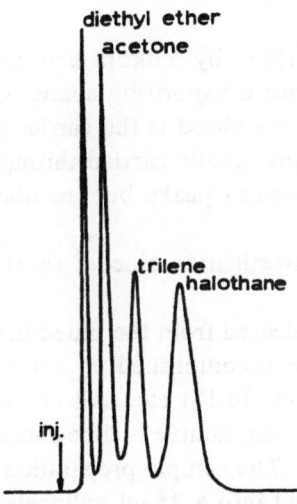

Fig. 5. Chromatogram of some organic anaesthetic agents and acetone.

the standard deviation of the peak height was less than 2%. The relationship between the concentration and the peak height is determined daily by means of standard solutions. The standard solutions are prepared by vaporising a small amount of liquid anaesthetic in an air-tight closed bottle. The relationship is linear for those concentrations relavent in anaesthesia.

It should be noted that analysis can be performed faster if only one organic anaesthetic is present.

ANALYSIS OF ORGANIC ANAESTHETIC AGENTS IN BLOOD
The concentration of volatile anaesthetic agents in blood can be determined in several ways. The result is obtained fastest if the blood is injected directly into the injection port (1, 4, 9-11). However, some problems arise which are not easily overcome.

If the temperature of the injection port is low, broad and asymmetrical peaks appear since the anaesthetic agent vaporises slowly and irregularly out of the blood. If the temperature of the injection port is high, clogging of the microsyringe and contamination of the column with protein material may occur (11). Furthermore, the amount of water which is introduced is rather large. Although water is not detected by a flame ionization detector it adversely affects the sensitivity of the detector. Separation of water and anaesthetic agents or removal of the water by means of absorption is necessary. In spite of the short total analysis time, direct injection of blood is not much used.

A similar method has been described by Yokota and co-workers (12). In this case the blood is injected into a vaporising space. Only when the anaesthetic has been released from the blood is the carrier gas introduced into the vaporising space and the anaesthetic carried through the column. This method produces more symmetrical peaks but the above mentioned objections still exist.

Both methods deserve further investigation since a short total analysis time is desirable.

In most cases the anaesthetic is released from the blood before the actual analysis is performed. This can be accomplished by extraction (10, 13), distillation (14-15), equilibration (1-4, 16-17) etc. All of these techniques have in common that preparation of the sample is time-consuming.

We use an equilibration method. The sample preparation is as follows: (Fig. 6) 400 μl of blood is introduced into a 25 ml volumetric flask, which

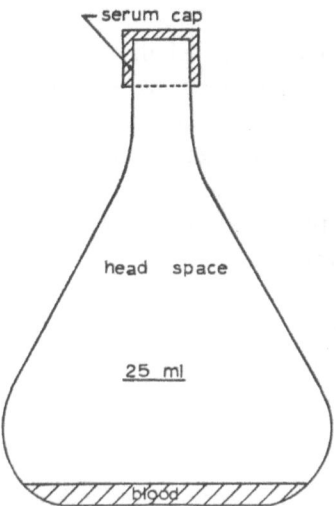

Fig. 6. Equilibration flask for analysis of anesthetic agaents in blood.

has been cut off at the graduation and closed with a serum cap. Then the flask is agitated for ten minutes in a shaker. In this time the halothane is distributed between the gas phase (head space) and the blood. Finally 200 μl of the gas phase is injected into the gas chromatograph.

The concentration of the halothane in the blood is determined from measurement of the peak height. The relationship between the peak height and the concentration is determined daily by means of standard solutions of halothane in blood (18). In normal cases the relationship is linear.

SAMPLING OF RESPIRATORY GASES

Halothane in respiratory gases is measured during anaesthesia or recovery by introducing 0.5 ml respiratory gas via a sample valve. In the sampling position (Fig. 7; 'membrane', unbroken line) one end of the sample loop is connected to the endotracheal tube. The connection is a 5 m stainless steel capillary tube (inner diameter 0.5 mm) joined at the patient's end to a 30 cm teflon tube (inner diameter 0.45 mm). The teflon tube is inserted into the endotracheal tube. The other end of the sample loop is connected to a vacuum system (pressure 0.37 kg/cm²). The dimensions of the transport tubes are such that negligible mixing occurs. The stainless steel tube is heated directly to prevent condensation of expired water vapour.

In this way gases are transported from the endotracheal tube to the vacuum system via the sample loop. Inspiratory and expiratory (alveolar) gases alternate in passing through the sample loop. If the sample loop is filled with expiratory gas, for example, the sample valve is brought into the injection position pneumatically (Fig. 7; 'membrane', broken line) and the sample is analysed by gas chromatography.

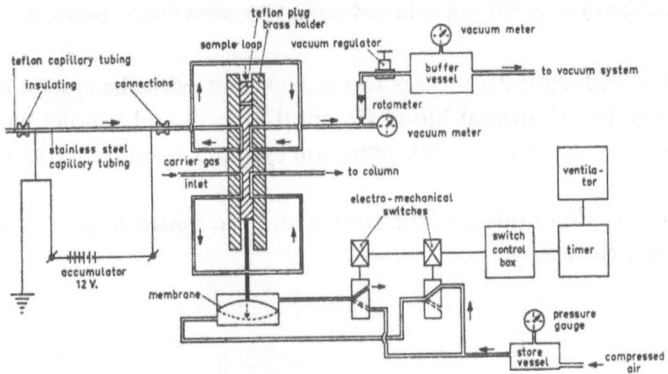

Fig. 7. System for sampling of respiratory gases.

Obviously the exact timing of the moment of injection is extremely important. In the event of artificial ventilation this is accomplished by a microswitch attached to the ventilator; this microswitch starts a delay timer which, after a pre-set time interval, in turn triggers the sampling valve. The exact time intervals which of course differ for inspiratory and expiratory gases are determined experimentally.

A detailed description of the system and the electronic circuits is in preparation.

RESULTS

These methods have been applied during a number of experiments to investigate the pharmacokinetics of halothane. Fig. 8 shows the results of some measurements carried out during recovery after a dog had been exposed to an inspiratory concentration of halothane of 0.94 vol % for 90 minutes.

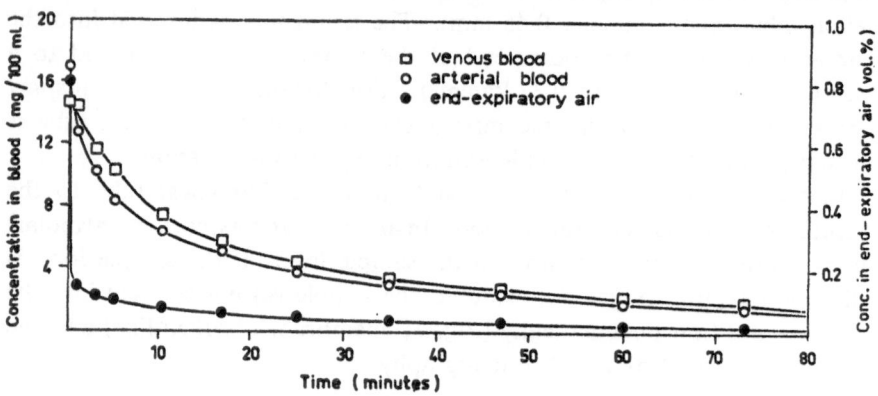

Fig. 8. Concentrations in blood and in end-expiratory gases during recovery.

Sampling of end-expiratory gases was carried out with the system described above. Samples of arterial blood (femoral artery) and venous blood (pulmonary artery) were drawn with precision syringes from the catheters in the arteries.

An extensive description of the results and the mathematical analysis will be published elsewhere.

REFERENCES

1. Weijer, W. F. P. M. van den, *Application of gas chromatography in anaesthesiology*, graduation report. Eindhoven University of Technology, 1970.
2. Doedens, A. J., *Gas chromatographic analysis of respiratory gases and anaesthetic agents in blood*, graduation report. Eindhoven University of Technology, 1971.
3. Ramakers, J. M., *Investigation of the pharmacokinetics of some organic anaesthetic agents by means of gas chromatography*, graduation report. Eindhoven University of Technology, 1971.
4. Burm, A. G. L., *Gas chromatographic analysis of halothane in respiratory gases and in blood*, graduation report. Eindhoven University of Technology, 1973.
5. Cramers, C. A. M. G. & Beneken Kolmer, H. H., Gas chromatography and anaesthesiology, *Chemisch Weekblad* 67, no 48, 26 november 1971.
6. Littlewood, A. B., *Gas chromatography, principles, techniques and applications*. New York 1962.
7. Purnell, H., *Gas chromatography*. New York 1962.
8. Gough, T. A. & Walker, E. A., Techniques in gas chromatography, choice of detectors. *The analyst* 95, 1 (1970).
9. Lowe, H. J., Flame ionization detection of volatile organic anesthetics in blood, gases and tissues. *Anesthesiology* 25, 808 (1964).
10. Douglas, R., Hill, D. W. & Wood, D. G. L., Methods for the estimation of blood halothane concentrations by gas chromatography. *Brit. J. Anaesth.* 42, 119 (1970).
11. Cousins, M. J. & Mazze, R. I., A rapid direct injection method for measuring volatile anesthetics in whole blood. *Anesthesiology* 36, 293 (1972).
12. Yokota, T., Hitomi, Y., Ohta, K. & Kosaka, F., Direct injection method for gas chromatographic measurement of inhalation anesthetics in whole blood. *Anesthesiology* 28, 1064 (1967).
13. Brachet–Liermain, A., Ferrus, L. & Caroff, J., Electron capture detection and measurement of fluothane (halothane) in blood. *J. chromatographic Sci.* 9, 49 (1971).
14. Dyferman, A. & Sjövall, J., Estimation of fluothane by gas chromatography. *Acta Anaesth. Scand.* 6, 171 (1962).
15. Gadsden, R. M., Risinger, B. H. & Bagwell, E. F., Determination of blood halothane levels by gas chromatography. *Can. Anaesth. Soc. J.* 12, 90 (1965).
16. Yamamura, H., Wakasugi, B., Sato, S. & Takebey, Y., Gas chromatographic analysis of inhalation anesthetics in whole blood by an equilibration method. *Anesthesiology* 27, 311 (1966).
17. Fink, B. R. & Morikawa, K., A simplified method for the measurement of volatile anesthetics in blood by gas chromatography. *Anesthesiology* 32, 451 (1970).
18. Cowles, A. L., Borgstedt, H. H. & Gillies, A. J., Solubilities of ethylene, cyclopropane, halothane and diethyl ether in human and dog blood at low concentrations. *Anesthesiology* 35, 203 (1971).

PART THREE

MEASUREMENT OF THE CIRCULATION

THE ASSESSMENT OF MYOCARDIAL FUNCTION

C. M. CONWAY

The prime function of the cardiovascular system is to supply blood to tissues and thereby provide an adequate amount of oxygen and remove adequate quantities of carbon dioxide and other waste products. The normal heart receives a venous return of blood from tissues – determined largely by tissue nutrient requirements – and expels the same volume back into the circulation. Intricate and complex mechanisms exist which enable the heart to act as a highly effective demand pump over a wide range of input volumes.

In a consideration of cardiac function it is convenient to analyse the various factors which affect cardiac output. Cardiac output is the product of heart rate and stroke volume, whilst stroke volume is the determinant of preload, afterload and the inotropic state of the heart (Fig. 1). The assessment of cardiac output is considered elsewhere in this book (p. 138), and this chapter is confined to a consideration of the influences of heart rate, preload, afterload and the inotropic state on myocardial performance.

CARDIAC   OUTPUT   =   STROKE   VOLUME   X   HEART   RATE

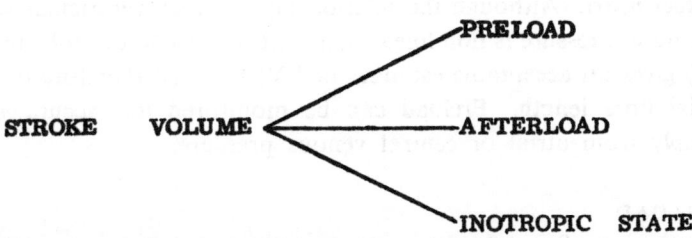

Fig. 1. The determinants of cardiac output.

1. HEART RATE

The heart rate is the most easily and most commonly measured variable of cardiac performance. The intrinsic rate due to normal action of the sinoatrial node is greatly influenced by central and peripheral factors. Thus measurements of pulse rate alone give little information as to the efficiency of cardiac function. In health, parasympathetic effects upon the S.A. node predominate and cardiac denervation normally causes an increase in heart rate. The chemically denervated heart in man has a rate in the order of 110 beats/min. Increases in heart rate normally increase cardiac output. As heart rate increases diastolic filling becomes progressively impaired, and at very high rates cardiac output will fall.

2. PRELOAD

This is a measure of initial myocardial fibre length. The relationship between initial fibre length and output is embodied in the Frank–Starling relationship – the greater the initial fibre length the more forcible is ventricular contraction. Preload is best measured as the left ventricular end-diastolic volume (LVEDV). This may be measured by cineangiography if assumptions are made on the geometry of the ventricle. Alternatively, if an indicator is injected into the ventricle and indicator concentration measured in outflowing blood as near to the ventricle as possible an indicator dilution curve made up of a series of steps can be recorded (Fig. 2). The ratios of the heights of successive steps gives the ratio of end-diastolic to end-systolic volumes. If stroke volume is determined from the area beneath the total washout curve, end-diastolic volume can also be assessed. This form of output curve is most easily obtained from the right side of the heart, using heat as the indicator and detecting temperature changes in the pulmonary artery. More recently the use of fibre-optic catheters has allowed dye concentrations during cardiac output determination to be measured just beyond the aortic valve. As ventricular volume is difficult to measure, preload is assessed from intracardiac pressure in most studies of function of the intact heart. Although the relationship between ventricular volume and transmural pressure is non-linear, left ventricular end-diastolic pressure (LVEDP) gives an acceptable estimate of LVEDV and therefore of initial myocardial fibre length. Preload can be monitored less accurately but more simply from atrial or central venous pressure.

3. AFTERLOAD

At the beginning of systole the ventricle contracts and pressure within it

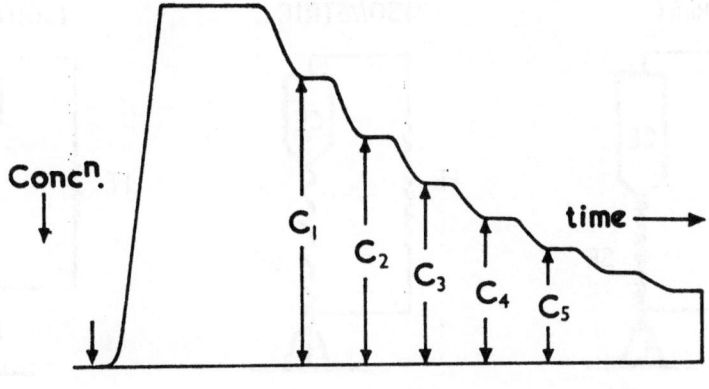

$$\frac{C_5}{C_4} = \frac{C_4}{C_3} = \frac{C_3}{C_2} = \frac{C_2}{C_1} = \frac{E.S.V.}{E.D.V.}$$

Fig. 2. End-diastolic volume estimation from rapid response dye dilution curves. The ratio of the heights of successive steps is equal to the ratios of end-systolic and end-diastolic volumes.

rises until intraventricular pressure exceeds aortic pressure. At this point the aortic valves open and ejection occurs. Blood is ejected into the arterial tree until aortic pressure exceeds that in the left ventricle. The amount of shortening of ventricular fibres and therefore the volume of blood ejected with each systole will be affected by the afterload imposed by aortic (or pulmonary) impedance. The higher the impedance the less blood will be ejected. Afterload is most commonly assessed as the mean arterial pressure.

4. INOTROPIC STATE

The inotropic state or "contractility" of cardiac muscle has been analysed by analogy with the skeletal muscle model of A. V. Hill (Fig. 3). This is a conceptual model which assumes that each fibre consists of a contractile element (CE) and a series elastic element (SE). An additional parallel elastic element (PE) is added to the original model to account for the resting diastolic tone of the cardiac muscle. Contraction occurs in two phases. Initially the CE contracts and stretches the SE, increasing tension within the fibre until the initial load on the muscle can be overcome. This isometric phase is followed by further shortening of the CE with no change

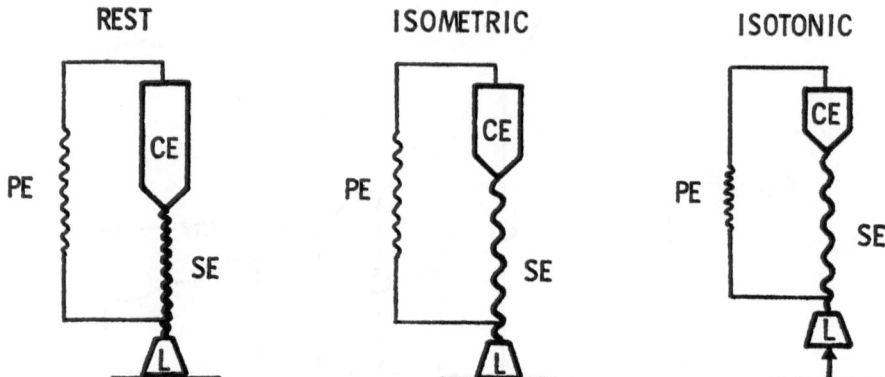

Fig. 3. Muscle model for the analysis of contractility.
CE – contractile element, SE – series elastic element,
PE – parallel elastic element, L – load.

in length of the SE and no change in tension – the phase of isotonic contraction. These two phases of muscle contraction correspond approximately to the isovolumic and ejection phases of ventricular systole.

Measurements of tension and length of an isolated papillary muscle can be made with the apparatus shown in Figure 4. The fibre M, attached at one end to a force transducer TT and at the other end to a lever, L, is stretched by a small initial preload, P, initial length being limited by a stop, S. A larger afterload, A, is then added and the fibre stimulated by electrodes E. Length and tension are recorded (Fig. 5), and by using different afterloads a series of curves are obtained (Fig. 6). From these curves the initial velocities of shortening at different loads can be obtained, and the force-velocity relations of the muscle under its specified conditions of contractility and preload may then be plotted (Fig. 7). Extrapolation of this curve to zero load gives the maximal velocity of shortening (V_{max}). Alteration in preload affects the slope of the force-velocity curve without affecting V_{max}. Exposure of the fibre to agents which increase inotropy, such as isoprenaline, displaces the whole curve with an increase in V_{max}.

In the intact heart a number of methods have been used to assess the contractile state indirectly. The best known of these is the measurement of the rate of change of pressure (dp/dt). In Fig. 8 simultaneous values of left ventricular pressure (LV) and dp/dt are shown. The maximum value of dp/dt occurs just before aortic valve opening. Increased inotropy is associated with increases in dp/dt max. However dp/dt max. is a complex function and is affected by changes in preload, afterload and heart rate (1).

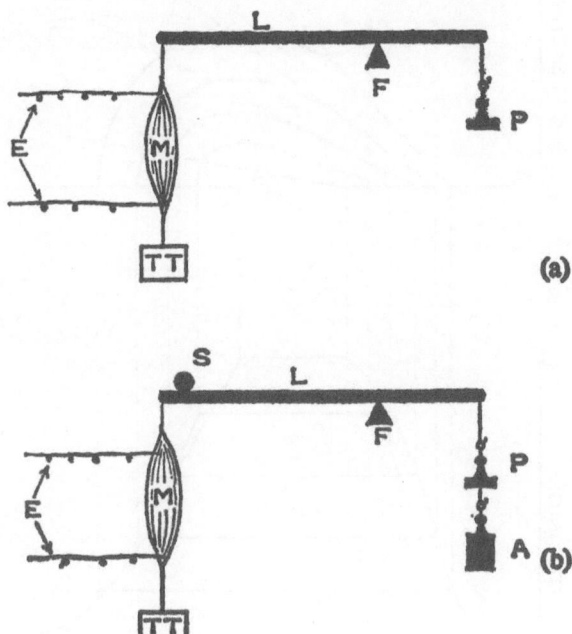

Fig. 4. Apparatus for the measurement of muscle mechanics. For explanation of symbols see text.

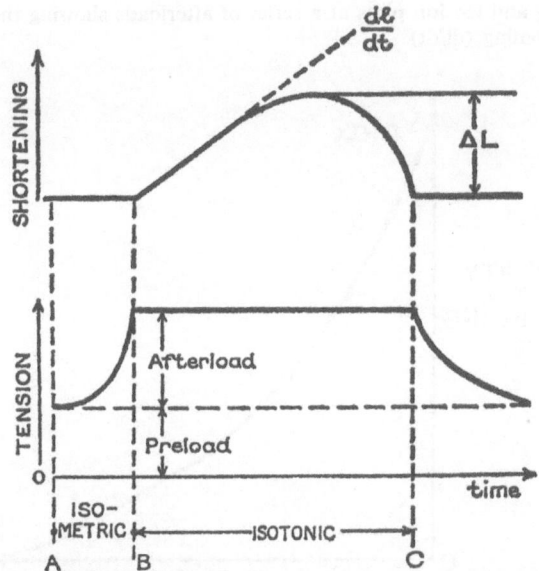

Fig. 5. Plots of shortening and tension against time for a single papillary muscle fibre.

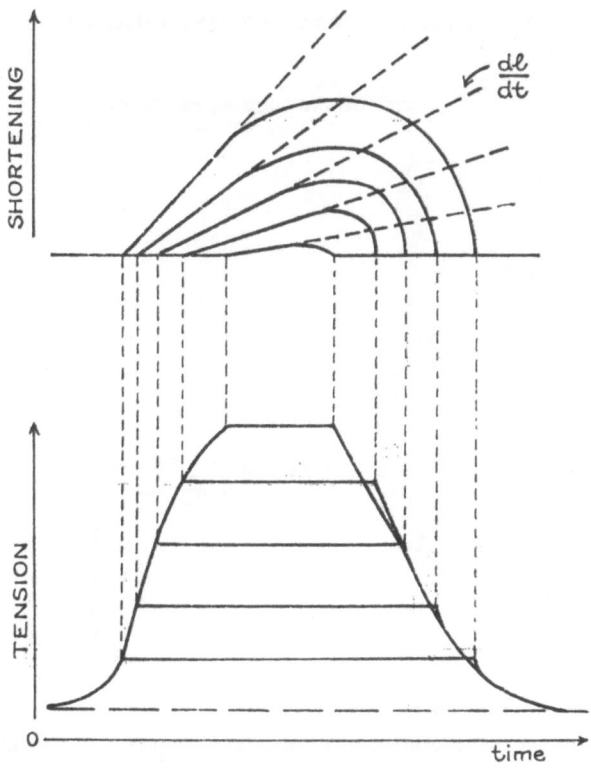

Fig. 6. Shortening and tension plots at a series of afterloads showing the various initial veloc ties of shortening (dl/dt).

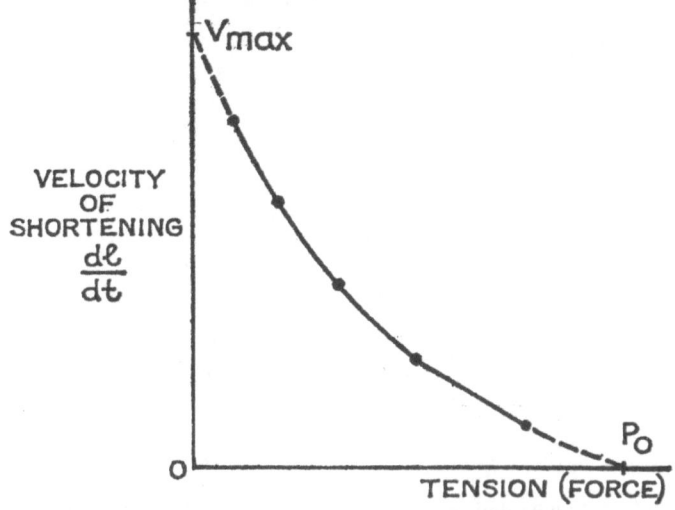

Fig. 7. Force velocity curve with extrapolation to V_{max} and P_o.

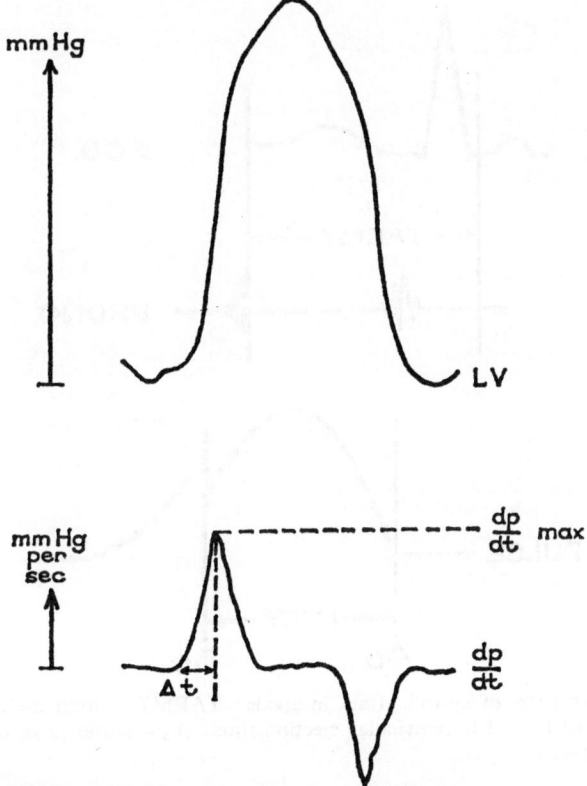

Fig. 8. Left ventricular pressure and its first derivative, dp/dt.

A more independent estimate of inotropy is given by the ratio of dp/dt_{max} to the developed pressure, by measuring the time to dp/dt_{max}, or by an indirect assessment of V_{max} by a continuous plot of dp/dt against isovolemic pressure and subsequent extrapolation (2). In experimental preparations where heart rate may be controlled by pacing and preload and afterload suitably kept constant, dp/dt_{max} may be used as a good estimate of the inotropic state (3). Measurements of dp/dt require the use of catheter-manometer systems with a high frequency response and either short rigid catheters or catheter-tip manometers must be used.

A somewhat similar measure of inotropy is the maximum aortic blood flow acceleration (4), which is largely independent of changes in preload, afterload and rate. This measurement has but rarely been made in man.

Because of the ease with which they can be obtained, measurements of

C. M. CONWAY

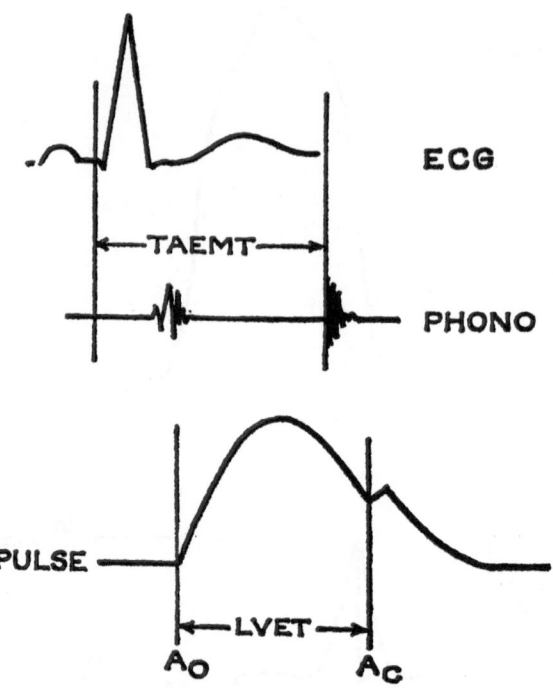

Fig. 9. The derivation of systolic time intervals. TAEMT – total active electro-mechanical time. LVET – left ventricular ejection time. A_o – aortic valve opening. A_c – aortic valve closure.

systolic time intervals are an attractive method of assessing the inotropic state of the heart. Simultaneous recordings of an ECG, phonocardiogram and an arterial pulse waveform are required to estimate total active electromechanical time, left ventricular ejection time and pre-ejection period (Fig. 9). Initial studies showed good correlation between the inverse of the pre-ejection period or its square (1/PEP or $1/PEP^2$) and other measures of inotropy over a wide range of experimental conditions. Under well controlled conditions PEP has been used to determine the effects of CO_2 upon the inotropic state of the heart (5) (Fig. 10). More recent studies in man have shown that PEP and its inverse derivatives are markedly sensitive to changes in preload (6). The ratio of pre-ejection period to left ventricular ejection time – PEP/LVET – has been widely used as a single expression of ventricular performance. Weissler and his colleagues (7) have reviewed the advantages and limitations of this ratio in the assessment of myocardial function in various pathological states.

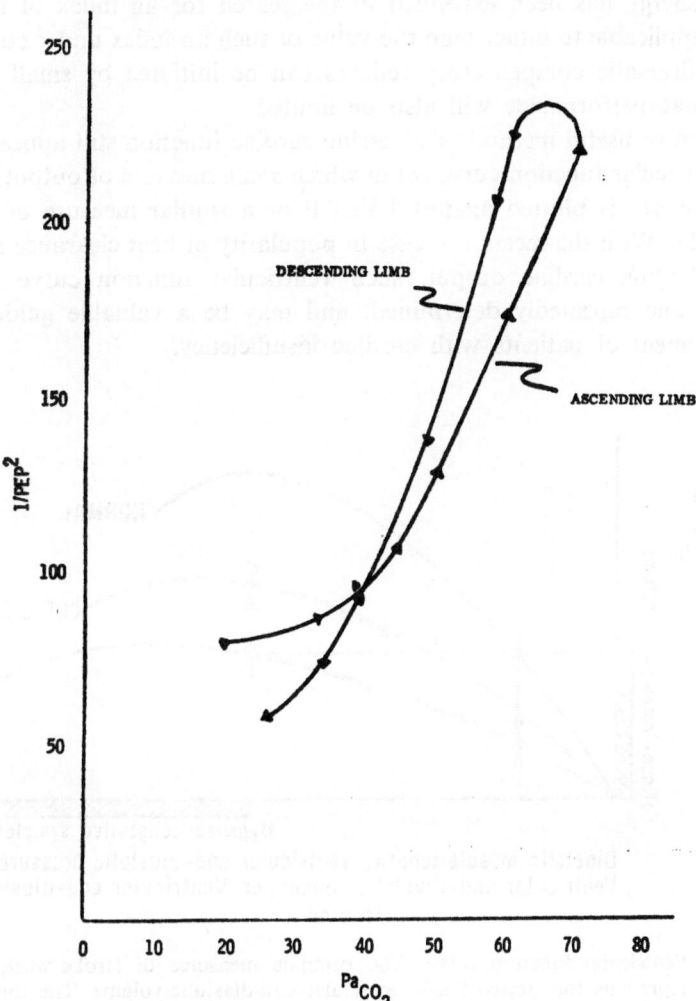

Fig. 10. Inotropy assessed by $1/PEP^2$ and Pa_{CO_2} in an anaesthetised patient at constant volume ventilation and varying arterial CO_2 tensions.

GENERAL ASSESSMENT OF CARDIAC FUNCTION
It is important to bear in mind that in the intact organism all factors affecting cardiac performance are interdependent, and little information is derived from a study of a single factor in isolation. Arterial pressure and heart rate are easily measured, but the limitations on information which can be derived from changes in these variables are well-known. Although

much energy has been expended in the search for an index of inotropy easily applicable to intact man the value of such an index under conditions where dramatic compensatory reflexes can be initiated by small changes in cardiac performance will also be limited.

The most useful method of assessing cardiac function still appears to be the ventricular function curve (8) in which some measure of output, usually stroke work, is plotted against LVEDP or a similar measure of preload (Fig. 11). With the recent increase in popularity of heat clearance methods of evaluating cardiac output, such ventricular function curves can be readily and repeatedly determined, and may be a valuable guide in the management of patients with cardiac insufficiency.

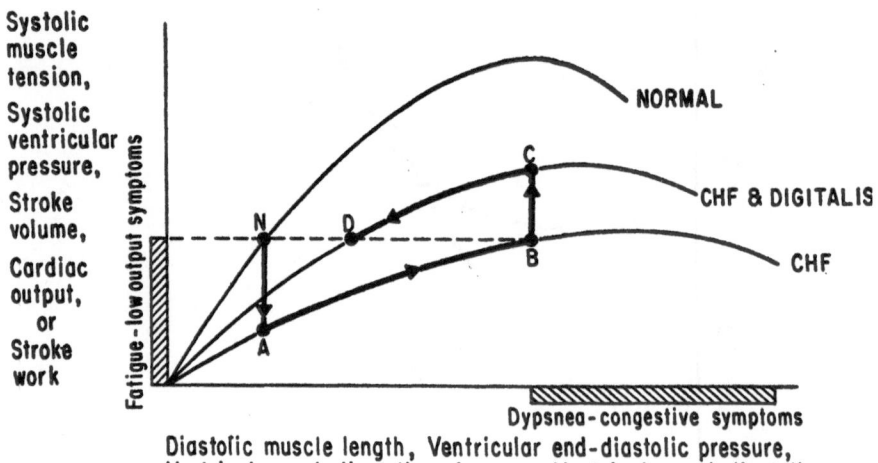

Fig. 11. Ventricular function curve. The ordinate measures of stroke work and the abscissa represents fnncttons of left ventricular end-diastolic volume. The three curves represent the normal heart, congestive heart failure and its treatment with digitalis. The sequence N-A-B-C-D shows depressed inotropy, Frank Starling compensation, restoration of inotropy with digitalis, and a reduction in the use of the Frank Starling mechanism.

(From Mason, D.T., Zelis, R., Amsterdam, A. and Massumi, R.A., Clinical determination of left ventricular contractility. In *Progress in Cardiology*, edited P.N. Yu and J.F. Goodwin, Leas and Febiger, Philadelphia, 1972, p. 121.

REFERENCES

1. Mason, D. T., Usefulness and limitations of the rate of rise of intraventricular pressure (dp/dt) in the evaluation of myocardial contractility in man. *Amer. J. Cardiol* 23, 516 (1969).
2. Shimosato, S., Isovolemic intraventricular pressure change: An index of myocardial contractility during Anesthesia. *Anesthesiology* 31, 327 (1969).
3. Furnival, C. M., Linden, R. J. & Snow, H. M., An assessment of the effect of the sympathetic nerves to the heart. *J. Physiol.* 191, 60P (1967).
4. Noble, M. I. M., Trenchard, D. and Guz, A., Left ventricular ejection in conscious dogs. *Circulat.* 19, 139 (1966).
5. Blackburn, J. P., Conway, C. M., Leigh, J. M., Lindop, M. J. & Reitan J. A., $Paco_2$ and the pre-ejection period – the $Paco_2$/inotropy response curve. *Anesthesiology* 37, 268 (1972).
6. Blackburn, J. P., Conway, C. M., Davies, R. M., Enderby, G. E. H., Edridge, A. W., Leigh, J. M., Lindop, M. J., Phillips, G. D. & Strickland, D. A. P., Valsava responses and systolic time intervals during anaesthesia and induced hypotension. *Brit. J. Anaesth.* 45, 704 (1973).
7. Weissler, A. M., Harris, W. S. & Schoenfeld, C. D., Bedside technics for the evaluation of left ventricular function in man. *Amer. J. Cardiol.* 23, 577 (1969).
8. Sarnoff, S. J., Myocardial contractility as defined by ventricular function curves. *Physiol. Rev.* 35, 107 (1955).

THE MEASUREMENT OF BLOOD FLOW
AND CARDIAC OUTPUT

P. CLIFFE

The present paper is a review of some of the methods of measuring blood flow and cardiac output which have been applied clinically.

THE ELECTROMAGNETIC FLOWMETER

The electromagnetic flowmeter, first described by Kolin (1936) is today one of the most widely used and satisfactory devices for the measurement of blood flow. Models are available from several commercial firms for the measurement particularly of arterial flow, both experimentally and during clinical surgery. In its 'cuffed' or noncannulated form horseshoe-like transducers may be fitted around an intact, exposed artery which may be of any size above about 2 mm diameter. Typical examples of flow probes are shown in figure 1.

An electrical output is provided which is:

1. Linearly related to the instantaneous volume flow.
2. Independent of the velocity profile provided this is symmetrical.
3. Equally sensitive to forward and reverse flows which are discriminated.
4. Of adequate frequency response.
5. Capable of averaging to provide mean flow readings.
6. Independent of the viscosity or density of the medium.

The principle is shown in figure 2 and depends on the laws of electromagnetic induction, first described by Faraday. When a conductor moves across the lines of flux between the poles of a magnet, an electromotive force (EMF) is induced in the conductor and is proportional to the rate of cutting flux lines. Blood is a conductor and when flowing at a steady rate, the EMF, generated in a direction mutually perpendicular to the flux and the axis of the artery, is directly proportional to the volume flow within it. The flow signal is also proportional to the strength of the magnetic flux, and provided the separation of the electrodes is fixed and they fit closely to the

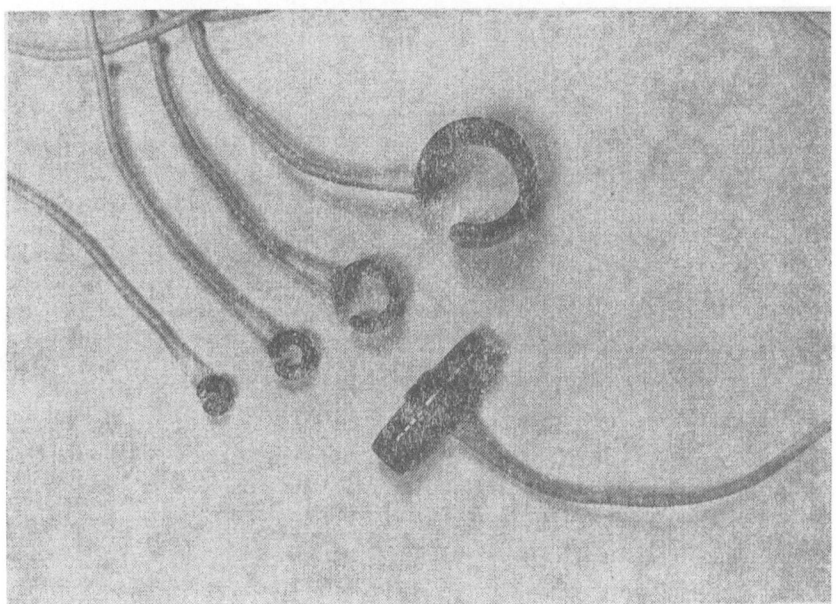

Fig. 1. Electromagnetic flow probes.

artery wall, the actual diameter of the vessel is not required.

The simple arrangement of a steady magnetic flux is not practicable, because a steady EMF would generate a direct current round the input circuit and polarisation at the electrodes would result. Consequently in modern electromagnetic flowmeters polarisation is avoided by the use of an alternating magnetic flux. In practice this is provided by an electromagnet supplied either with a sinusoidal or square wave current. The latter is alternately switched first in one direction and then in the other. Typical frequencies of the alternating supplies are approximately 400 Hz.

The use of alternating supplies gives rise to certain electronic problems. Thus reference to figure 2 shows that if the magnetic flux varies within the loop joining the electrodes to the input circuit, an EMF will be generated which is independent of the flow signal and would be present even though the blood were at rest. Various circuits have been employed to eliminate these additionally induced EMFs and the flow signal may be recovered for display and recording.

Typical magnet energizing current waveforms are shown in figure 3. In earlier instruments although the blood flow waveform could be satisfactorily recorded, instability in the zero was a problem. By using the pulsed magnet

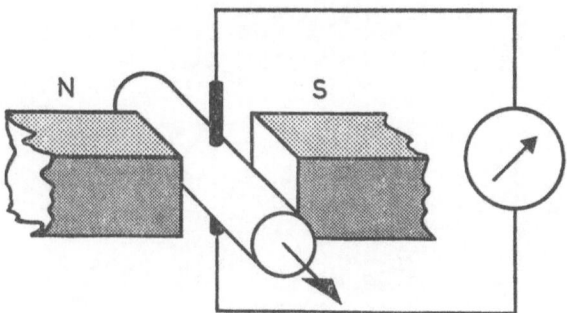

Fig. 2. Electromagnetic flow principle.

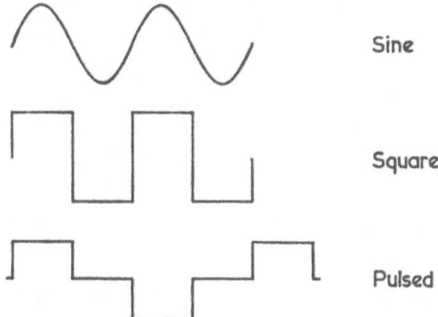

Sine

Square

Pulsed

Fig. 3. Magnet energisation waveforms.

energization, the current zeros between pulses allow the flow zero to be automatically corrected.

Figure 4 shows a comparison of the flow zero and electrical zero for a currently available commercial flowmeter using a cuffed probe applied to the femoral artery of a pig.

Electromagnetic flowmeters are finding increasing use during peripheral vascular surgery. Figure 5 shows the results obtained during the relief of carotid artery stenosis. This procedure may be carried out using a cervical plexus block and the state of conciousness of the patient may be assessed during manipulations on the internal carotid artery.

Figure 6 shows a Williams–Barefoot probe. This is a flexible electromagnetic flow probe developed for measuring aortic flow velocity, stroke volume and cardiac output following cardiac surgery. The flexible probe is fitted around the aortic root, prior to chest closure, held with a suture and brought out through the chest incision. By integrating the flow signal, stroke volume

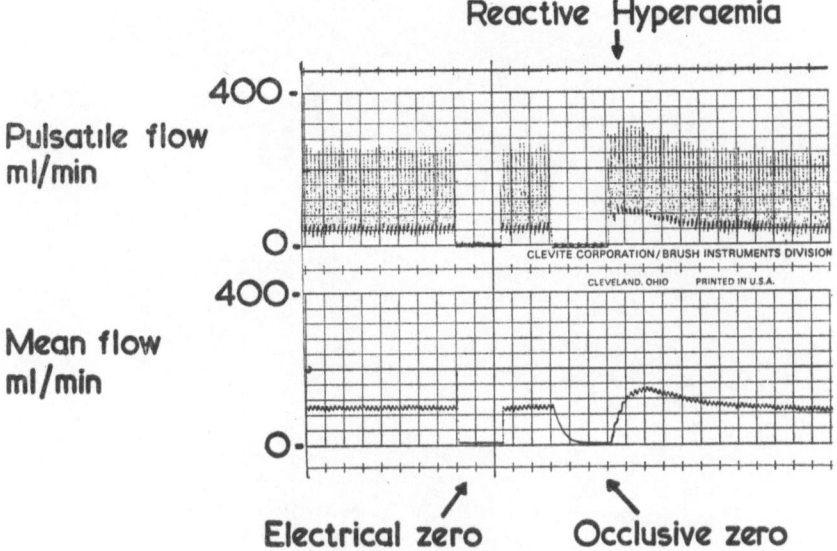

Fig. 4. Comparison of electrical and occlusive zeros.

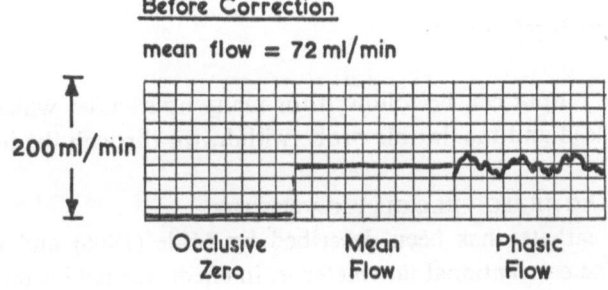

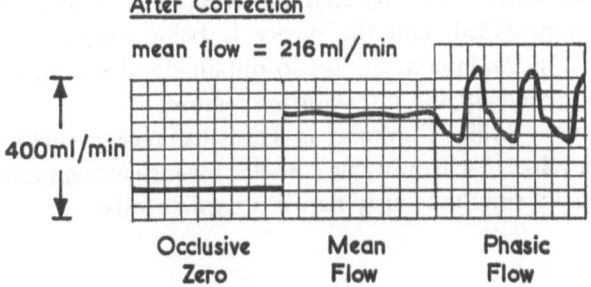

Fig. 5. Blood flow in carotid artery stenosis.

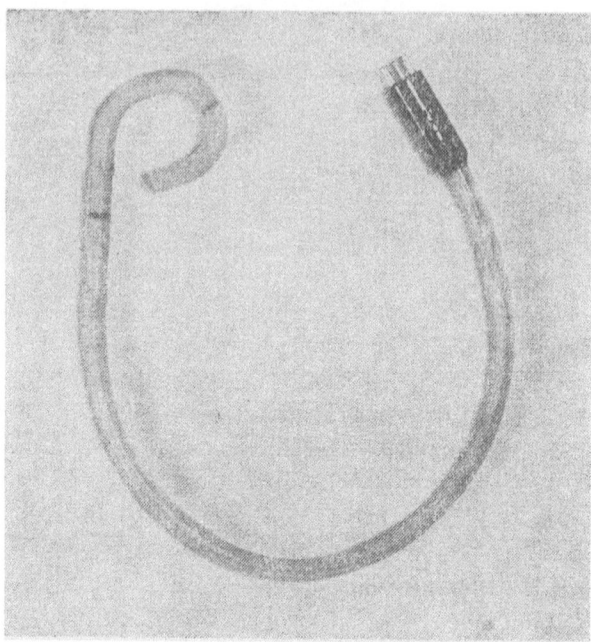

Fig. 6. Williams-Barefoot probe.

and cardiac output can be followed for many hours after which the suture can be released and the flexible probe withdrawn through the incision.

ELECTROMAGNETIC VELOCITY CATHETER
A velocity catheter has been described by Mills (1966) and is shown in figure 7. The conventional flowmeter is, in effect, turned inside out. A coil is wound at the end of a No. 6 cardiac catheter and the passage of current produces a magnetic flux inside the vessel. Electrodes are mounted in the catheter across which a velocity signal is generated. A pressure measuring lumen is also provided, and the device is being applied during cardiac catheterisation in the human subject to obtain simultaneous measurements of aortic blood velocity and intra-aortic pressure.
More recently the Millar Company in Texas has incorporated two pressure sensors and a velocity sensor in one catheter for measuring pressure gradient and flow velocity simultaneously across a cardiac valve.

THERMAL PROBES
Various thermal devices have been described for the measurement of blood

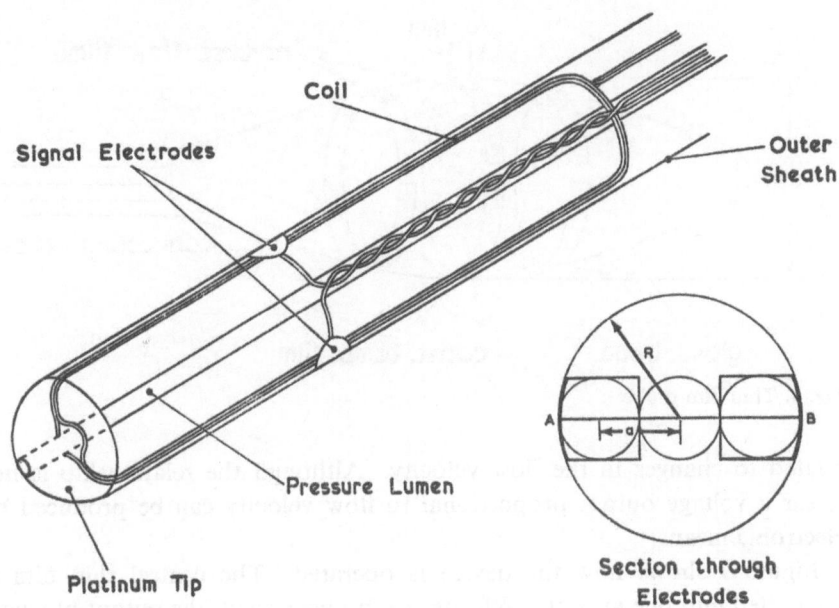

Coil

Signal Electrodes

Outer
Sheath

R

A
a
B

Pressure Lumen

Platinum Tip

Section through
Electrodes

Fig. 7. Velocity catheter.

flow in arteries and veins and also in tissues and organs. One of the earliest
was the thermostromuhr of Rein described in physiology texts.

Mellander and Rushmer (1960) described a thermal flowmeter applicable
to venous blood flow. While Hensel et al. (1961), Grayson (1952) and
Mowbray (1959) have shown how thermal probes in needle form may be
applied to blood flow in organs and tissues.

THIN FILM FLOWMETER
Considerable advances in thermal flow techniques have been achieved by
Shultz et al. (1969) who have applied the methods of thin film anemometry
to develop flow catheters and needles. In a typical probe, figure 8, the
thermal element consists of a glass bead 0.5 mm diameter onto which three
thin metallic films, approximately 1 micron in thickness, are deposited.
The central film acts as a resistance thermometer which allows the surface
temperature to be determined, and simultaneously as a heating element to
heat the bloodstream.

The film is maintained at a constant temperature a few degrees centigrade
above the surroundings when variation in the electrical power supply are

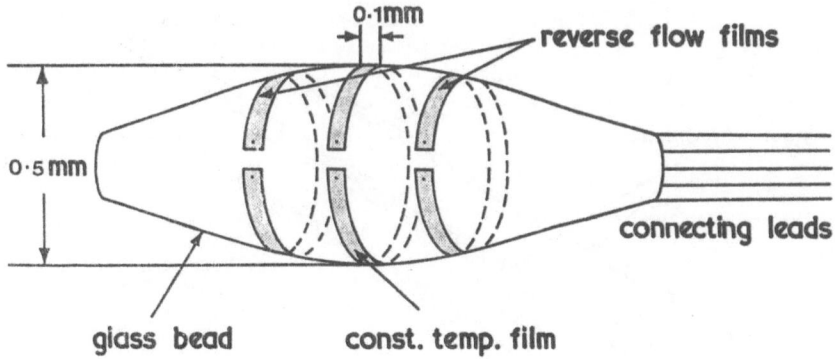

Fig. 8. Thin film probe.

related to changes in the flow velocity. Although the relationship is not linear a voltage output proportional to flow velocity can be produced by electronic means.

Figure 9 shows how the device is operated. The central thin film is connected into one arm of a Wheatstone bridge circuit, the output of which is fed into a D.C. amplifier. The amplifier output is fed back to the bridge supply in such a way that as the temperature of the thin film tends to fall, more power is supplied to the bridge.

The device has a sufficiently rapid response to demonstrate turbulence in the circulation. A disadvantage of such a probe, if only the central film were provided, would be its inability to detect flow reversal. Clearly it is

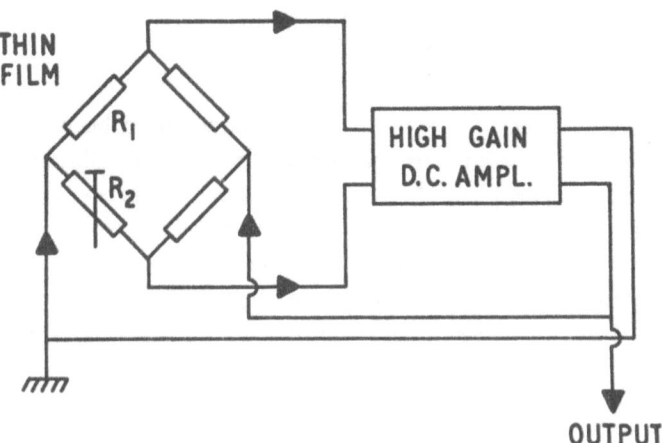

Fig. 9. Constant temperature circuit.

immaterial as regards heat transfer whether the flow is upstream or down-stream.

The other two films are therefore provided to detect flow direction. Thus blood flowing from the constant temperature film to the lefthand film will heat it, whereas the righthand film is unaffected. The opposite conditions apply with flow reversal. Hence if the two outer films form adjacent arms of a Wheatstone bridge, the output will vary on one side of zero or the other depending on the flow direction. Thin film probes have been applied in man and in the experimental animal. Figure 10 shows the flow pattern in aortic stenosis. At operation, the distribution of velocities was examined along an aortic diameter. The region of the jet of blood through the stenosis could be outlined. The very high jet velocity of about 250 cm/sec., with turbulence within the jet, is clearly apparent. The normal peak aortic flow velocity is of the order of 80 cm/sec. and is non-turbulent in the experimental animal, at rest.

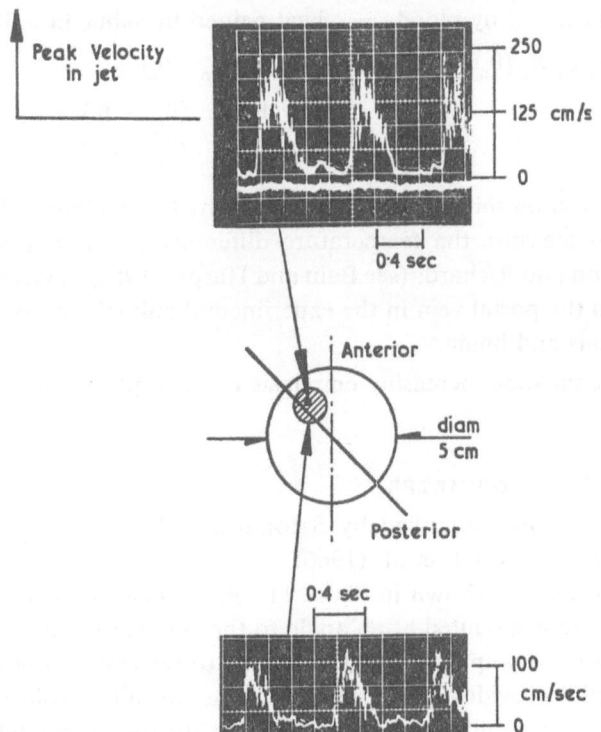

Fig. 10. Velocity measurements in aortic stenosis.

LOCAL THERMAL DILUTION

Warm or cold saline may be injected into a blood vessel and the temperature of the blood-saline mixture is measured with a thermistor or thermocouple mounted in a catheter a few centimetres downstream. Suppose the flow is undirectional and that adequate mixing occurs, and the temperature sensing device has an adequate response time.

If
$\dot{Q}$ = average blood flow, ml/sec.
$\dot{q}$ = saline injection rate, ml/sec.
θ_b = blood temperature before injection
θ_s = temperature of the injectate
θ_m = temperature of the blood/saline mixture
$d_b\, d_s$ = respective densities of blood and saline
$S_b\, S_s$ = respective specific heats of blood and saline

Then if no heat is lost or gained overall

heat lost by blood = heat gained by saline in unit time

i.e.
$$\dot{Q}\, d_b\, S_b\, (\theta_b - \theta_m) = \dot{q}\, d_s\, S_s\, (\theta_m - \theta_s)$$

∴
$$\dot{Q} = \dot{q} \cdot \frac{d_s\, S_s}{d_b S_b} \cdot \frac{(\theta_m - \theta_s)}{(\theta_b - \theta_m)} \tag{1}$$

A catheter based on this method was devised by Clark (1966). Thermistors were used to measure the temperature differences. The device has been used by Cotton and Richards (see Bain and Harper, 1968) to measure venous blood flow in the portal vein in the experimental animal and to splenic vein flow in animals and humans.

At the present time increasing emphasis is being placed on non invasive techniques.

DOPPLER SHIFT FLOWMETER

This device was first described by Satomura and Kaneko (1960) and an improved form by Stegall et al. (1966).

The arrangement is shown in figure 11. A piezoelectric crystal operated at about 5 MHz is mounted at an angle to the skin surface and driven by a power oscillator. By applying a suitable jelly to the skin a continuous path for ultrasound is provided. After reflection from the intermediate structures, and the blood vessel, ultrasound is received at the second crystal. In particular blood cells, which are moving, reflect the sound with a change in

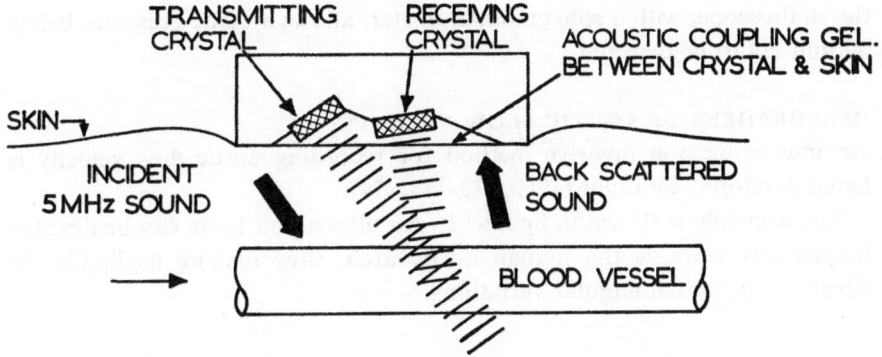

Fig. 11. Doppler shift flowmeter.

frequency. For a 5 MHz source the difference frequency is in the audible range being 6-7,000 Hz for blood velocities of about 100 cm/sec.

The pitch of the frequency deviation is proportional to the average instantaneous flow velocity. In several commercial instruments the audio frequency signal drives a loudspeaker and a note of varying pitch is heard when the transducer is placed over an artery. By converting frequency into a voltage proportional to amplitude the average instantaneous flow velocity may be recorded graphically.

The Doppler shift flowmeter has the advantage of direct application to the intact skin, but this is associated with some disadvantages. Thus the amplitude of the flow signal varies considerably with changes in the angle between the axis of the transducer and that of the blood vessel. Nevertheless the device is proving to be valuable clinically. For example, with practice it is possible to obtain a reasonable estimate of blood flow through peripheral arteries, and combined with selective angiography the flowmeter gives useful indications of the advisability of peripheral vascular surgery. It is being increasingly employed in the detection of postoperative venous thrombosis. If the flow transducer is directed towards the femoralvein, and the thigh is squeezed, or if the foot is dorsiflexed, the extra venous blood drained through the vein gives rise to a considerably enhanced sound, in absence of venous obstruction. By locating the transducer at various levels along the limb the approximate site of thrombosis may be demonstrated.

Another application concerns the measurement of systolic pressure under conditions of extreme hypotension. Using the ultrasonic probe instead of

the stethoscope, with a sphygmomanometer, allows systolic pressures below
50 mm Hg to be detected.

MEASUREMENT OF AORTIC FLOW VELOCITY
An interesting non invasive method for recording aortic flow velocity is
being developed by Light (1969, '72, '73, '74).

The principle is shown in figure 12. An ultrasound beam can be directed
tangentially towards the human aortic arch, thus making negligible the
effect of substantial angular variations.

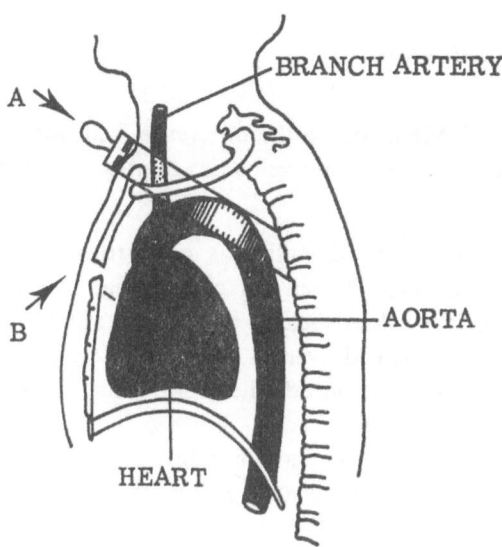

Fig. 12. Aortic flow velocity.

Quantitatively velocity measurement is possible if the angle θ between the
ultrasonic beam and the direction of flow is small. Thus the flow velocity
u is given by

$$u = \frac{k \cdot \Delta f}{\cos \theta} \qquad (2)$$

where Δf =   observed Doppler shift
          θ   =   angle between flow direction and ultrasonic beam
          k   =   constant for a particular instrument and depends on
                  its operating frequency.

If θ is less than 25° it is found that the flow velocity may be measured to within ± 5%.

The Doppler shift present at any time may be displayed by spectral analysis as shown in figure 13. The different frequencies between the transmitted and reflected ultrasound provides a spectrum within the audible range whose frequencies are proportional to the flow velocities. The outputs from eighteen audio filters are recorded on a paper chart, as a plot of instantaneous velocity versus time. Assuming a flat velocity profile within the aorta and measuring its diameter radiologically, integration of the velocity-time graph yields stroke volume and hence cardiac output.

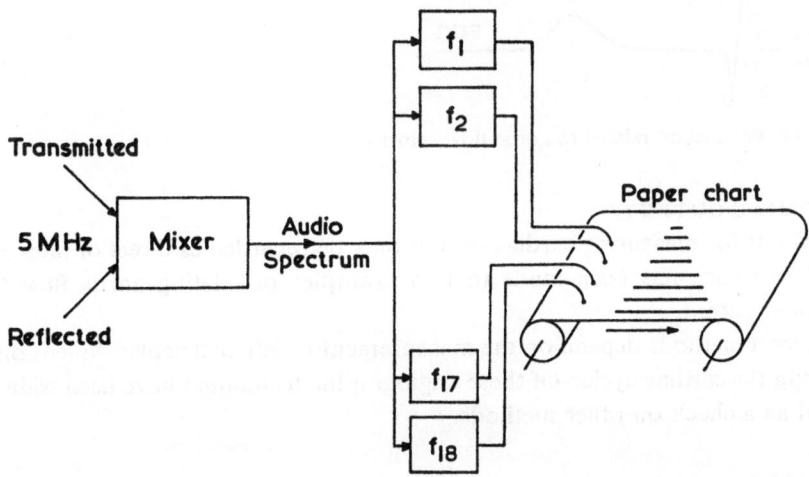

Fig. 13. Spectrum analyser.

Figure 14 shows diagrammatically the velocity time plot in relation to the electrocardiogram and shows additional factors may be derived and related to myocardial function.

The method is being correlated by Light and his coworkers with other methods of measuring cardiac output. The device has also been applied during surgery to follow aortic velocity during the administration of halothane anaesthesia. In one instance, following the reduction of halothane the blood pressure recovered fairly rapidly but the aortic blood flow returned only slowly to the pre-operative level.

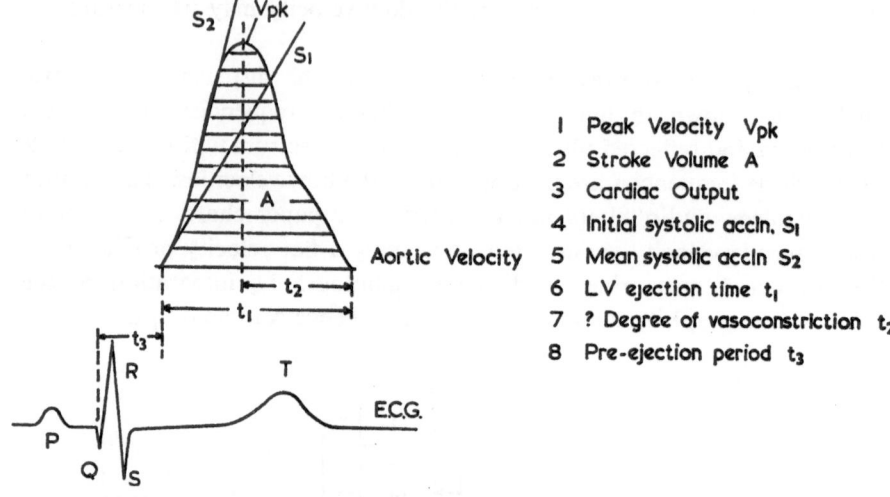

Fig. 14. Parameters related to aortic flow velocity.

CARDIAC OUTPUT

Methods for measuring cardiac output may be regarded as direct or indirect and reference has been made to two examples of relating aortic flow to cardiac output.

Direct methods depend on the measurement of left ventricular dimensions during the cardiac cycle. Of these angiographic techniques have been widely used as a check on other methods.

ANGIOGRAPHIC METHODS

The principles were eluciated by Dodge in 1960, who used biplane angiography. The situation is represented in figure 15. He pointed out that the left ventricular shadow in the A-P and lateral films was distorted by two factors, namely, the divergency of the X-ray beams and the orientation of the heart in space.

It was assumed that the L.V. cavity was an ellipsoid and that apex to aortic valve distance was its long axis. Suppose this distance is PQ in figure 15. Distances $P_1 Q_1$ and $P_2 Q_2$ are first corrected for orthogonal projection on their respective films. By resolving these corrected lengths along the x, y and z axes. The length and direction of PQ in space can be calculated.

To find the short axis of the ellipsoid the actual area of the L.V. shadow is measured on each film and from this the two short axes can be calculated.

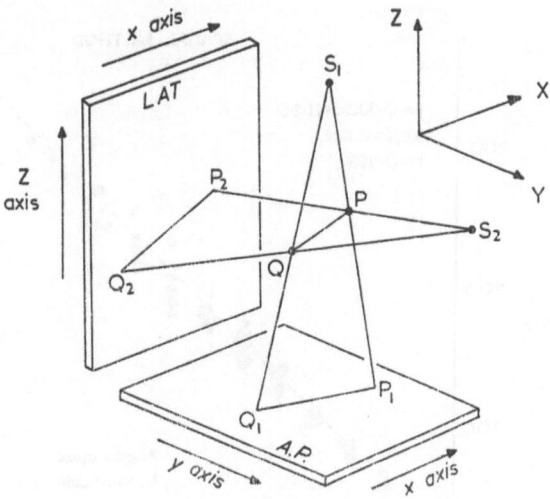

Fig. 15. Ventricular volumes by biplane angiography.

These lengths are also corrected for X-ray divergency and spatial position and hence the L.V. volume can be calculated. Thus if

$$L \quad = \quad \text{apex to aortic valve distance}$$
$$d_1 \, d_2 \quad = \quad \text{respective minor axes}$$

$$\text{L. V. volume} = \frac{4\pi}{3} \cdot \frac{L}{2} \cdot \frac{d_1}{2} \cdot \frac{d_2}{2} \qquad (3)$$

In testing the method Dodge X-rayed cadaver hearts containing contrast medium and also models of known volume and a high correlation resulted from the actual values and those calculated from angiography, as in figure 16. By measuring end systolic volume and end diastolic volume the stroke volume and hence the cardiac output can be derived if the pulse rate is known.

Later workers (Green et al. 1967, Sandler et al. 1968) have shown that a single right anterior oblique film is sufficient and recently a computer assisted method has been described by Marcus (1972) for analysing cineangiograms taken at 60 frames/sec. A disadvantage of the method is that it cannot be readily repeated.

ECHOCARDIOGRAPHY

Considerable progress has been made in recent years in the ultrasonic

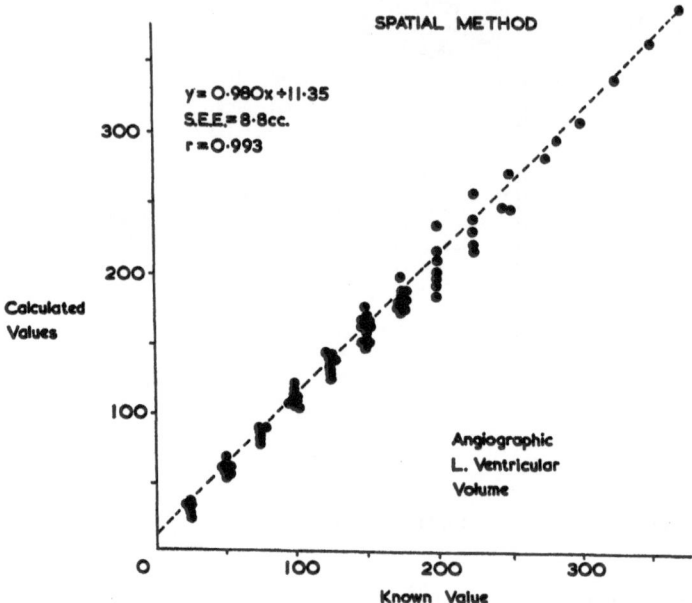

Fig. 16. Correlation between angiographic and actual volumes.

scanning of the heart. In 1969 it was shown that the transverse dimension of the left ventricle could be measured by echocardiography as the distance between echoes from the endocardial surfaces of the interventricular septum and the posterior wall (Chapelle and Mensch 1969, Feigenbaum et al. 1969).

When compared with the angiographic method this distance compares with the mean minor axis of the left ventricular ellipsoid. Hence in formula (3) above, if the echo distance

$$d = d_1 = d_2$$

and

$$2d = L$$

substitution yields

$$\text{L.V. volume} = \frac{4\pi}{3} \cdot \frac{2d}{2} \cdot \frac{d}{2} \cdot \frac{d}{2}$$

$$= \frac{\pi}{3} \cdot d^3 \tag{4}$$

i.e. the 'echo' volume is closely related to the cube of the echo dimension.

Figure 17 (Feigenbaum 1973) shows the principal scan paths which are

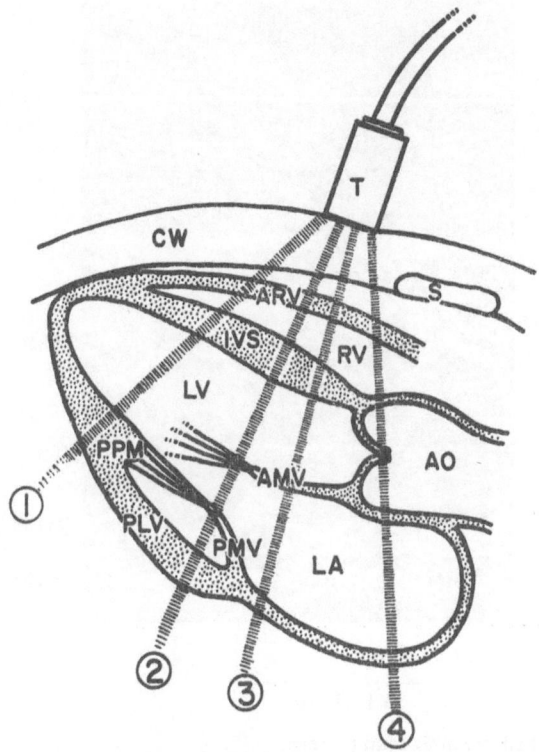

Fig. 17. Cardiac scan paths using ultrasound.

generally used and the second path is suitable for L.V. dimensions. The repeated echoes returning to the transducer build up a picture of the changing shape of the heart along the direction of the scan. Gibson (1973) has illustrated a typical scan shown in figure 18. The picture is automatically calibrated for distance vertically and time horizontally. The interventricular septum and the posterior left ventricular wall are identified. The end diastolic measurement is made on the R wave of the electrocardiogram, before slight movement associated with isovolumetric contraction, and end systolic measurement is at the time of the least separation of the two echoes. Hence the echo distance and its variation with time may be derived.

Gibson (1973) has correlated the echo and angiographic methods for end systolic and end diastolic volumes and the results are shown in figure 19. Clearly if the heart rate is also known the cardiac output can be calculated from the non-invasive echo measurements. Figure 20 illustrates a correlation

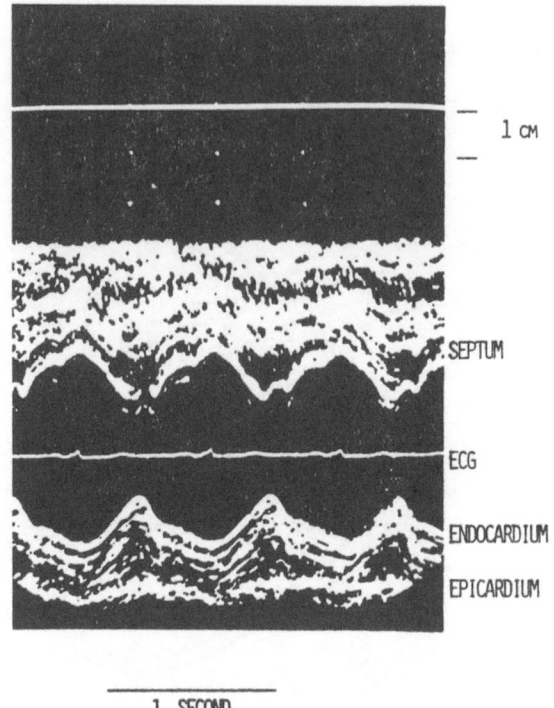

Fig. 18. Echocardiographic scan pattern.

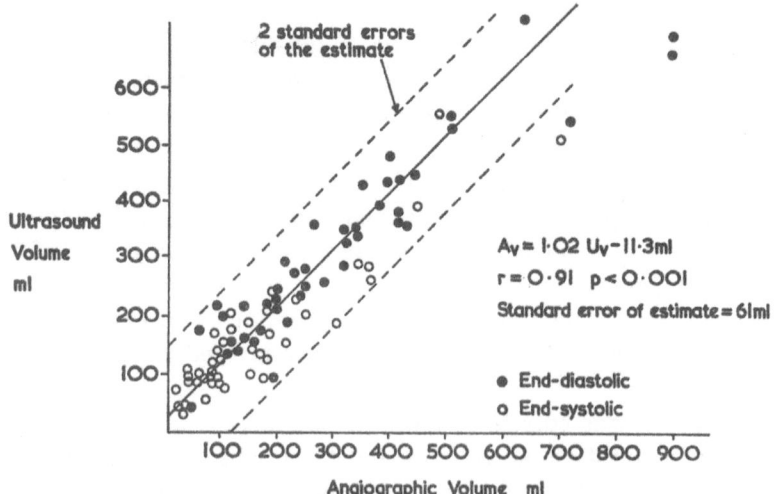

Fig. 19. Correlation between angiographic and ultrasonic ventricular volumes.

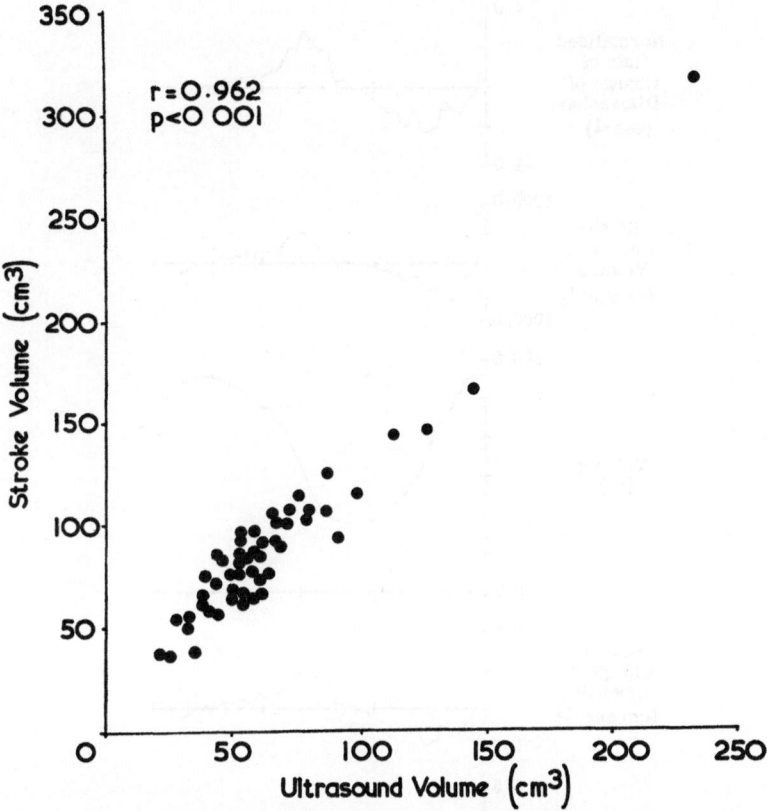

Fig. 20. Correlation between dye dilution and echographic stroke volumes.

(Feigenbaum 1973) between the echo stroke volume and that measured by dye dilution techniques.

Echocardiography is being further developed to yield valuable information about ventricular function. Thus Gibson (1974) has digitized the echocardiogram dimension and applied automatic analyses as shown in figure 21. This shows left ventricular dimension and rate of change from a patient with mitral regurgitation. Zero time is coincident with the inscription of the QRS complex of the electrocardiogram. An estimate of left ventricular volume as the cube of the dimension and its rate of change is also shown. This rate, during diastole is related to inflow into the L.V. and during systole to outflow via the aortic valve.

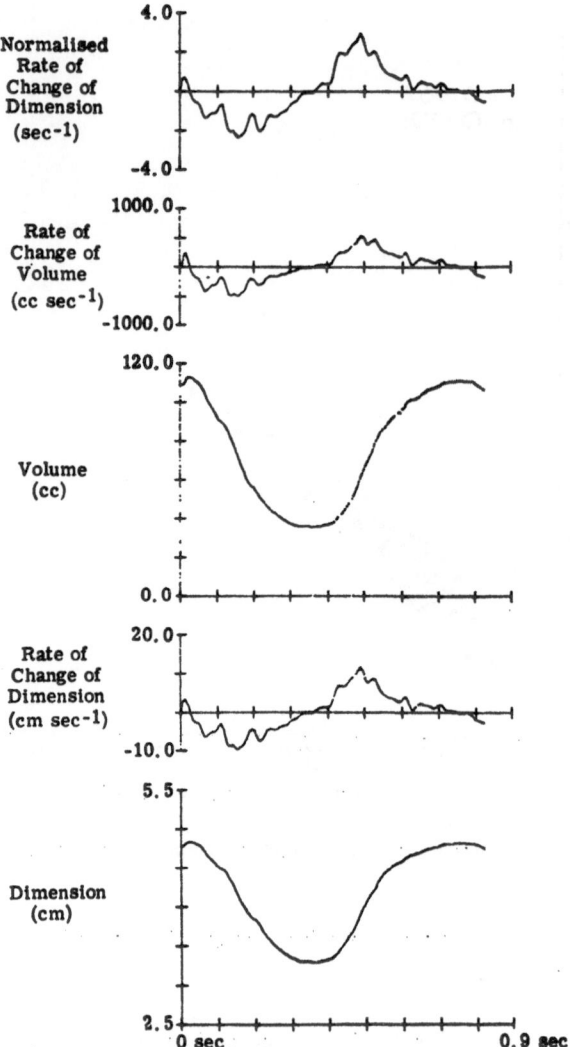

Fig. 21. Factors derived from echo dimension.

INDICATOR DILUTION TECHNIQUES

If an indicator substance is injected at a point in the circulation and its change of concentration with time is measured at a point downstream the flow rate along the pathway can be calculated.

This is the basis of the Fick method (1970) in which the indicator is a physiological substance, namely oxygen or carbon dioxide. Fick states that

$$\text{Cardiac Output} = \frac{\text{Rate of } O_2 \text{ uptake}}{C_a - C_v} \qquad (5)$$

where C_a and C_v are respectively the arterial and venous blood oxygen content. This relation is obvious with a simple example. For if the

$$\text{arterial content} = 18 \text{ vol } \% = 180 \text{ ml } O_2/\text{litre blood}$$
$$\text{venous} \quad \text{,,} \quad = 13 \text{ vol } \% = 130 \text{ ml } O_2/\text{litre blood}$$

then each litre of blood carries 50 ml O_2. If the rate of uptake is 250 ml O_2/min this must be carried by 5l of blood in each minute, which is the cardiac output.

DYE DILUTION METHODS

Non physiological indicators have been widely used for decades, and the one most commonly employed today is indocyanine green. It is detected photometrically at a wavelength of 800 nm which is an isobestic point for reduced and oxygenated haemoglobin.

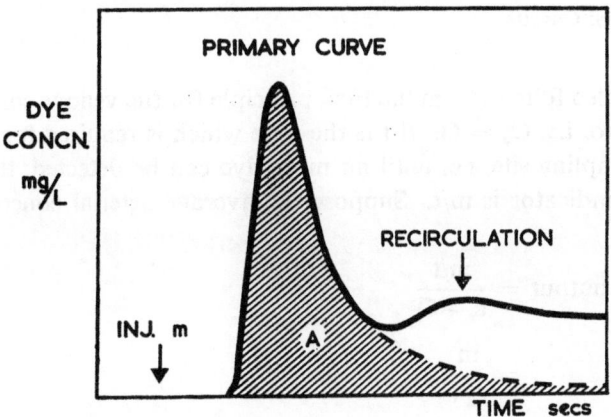

Fig. 22. Normal dye dilution curve.

Figure 22 shows a typical dye dilution curve obtained by drawing blood through a cuvette (figure 23) and recording the time concentration curve resulting from the photometric analysis. If the exponential downslope of the curve is projected to eliminate recirculation, the cardiac output is given, using the correct units, by the dye dose m divided by the extrapolated area A. If the dye concentration is expressed in mg/L and the time in seconds the area is mg.sec/L and the cardiac output will be in L/sec.

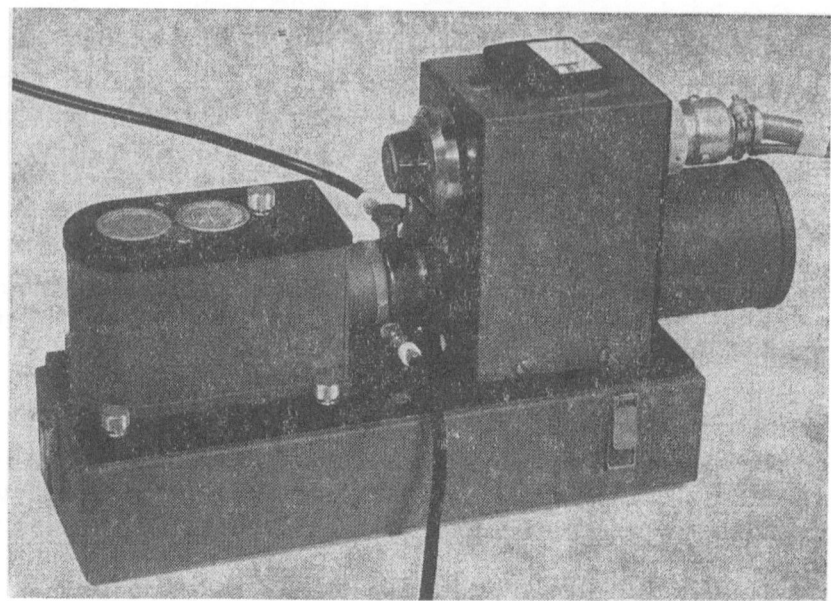

Fig. 23. Gilford Cuvette.

This result also follows from the Fick principle for the venous concentration of dye is zero, i.e. $C_v = O$. If t is the time which is required for the dye to pass the sampling site, i.e. until no more dye can be detected, then rate of passage of indicator is m/t. Suppose the average arterial concentration is c_a, then

the cardiac output $= \dfrac{m/t}{c_a - O}$

$= \dfrac{m}{c_a\, t}$

But the c_a is the average height of the curve and t is the 'length' of its base ∴ c_a t represents the area A and output = Dye dose/Area A.

THERMAL DILUTION
Another indicator which has become popular in recent years is provided by the heat content within the circulation for the production of thermal dilution curves. Typically 10 ml of dextrose at room temperature are injected into the right atrium and the temperature change in the pulmonary artery is recorded. This has exactly the same form as the dye curve but without

recirculation. The cardiac output is given by the 'heat dose' divided by the area under the curve just as for other dilution techniques. Thus if

$$V = \text{volume}$$
$$D = \text{density}$$
$$S = \text{specific heat}$$
$$\text{suffix } i = \text{injectate}$$
$$\text{suffix } b = \text{blood}$$
$$t = \text{time for cooled blood to be detected at the sampling site}$$
$$\Theta_b = \text{initial temperature in PA}$$
$$\Theta_i = \text{temperature of injectate}$$
$$\Delta\bar{\Theta} = \text{average temperature change}$$

$$\text{then cardiac output} = \frac{V_i \, D_i \, S_i \, (\Theta_b - \Theta_i)}{D_b \cdot S_b \cdot \Delta\bar{\Theta} \cdot t} \qquad (6)$$

However, heat content change in a system is given by the product of mass, specific heat and temperature change.

Thus as $V_i \, D_i$ is the mass injected the numerator of equation (6) is the 'heat dose'. Similarly $D_b = \dfrac{M_b}{V_b}$ and hence $D_b \, S_b \, \Delta\bar{\Theta}$ is the average heat change during time t divided by the volume of blood passing in that time i.e. the 'average heat concentration'. Hence the denominator of equation (6) is the area under the temperature time graph multiplied by the constants D_b and S_b.

Thermal dilution methods have been correlated with the Fick method by Branthwaite and Bradly (1968) and figure 24 has been redrawn from their results.

Computers are now available for integrating dye curves and similar devices for thermal curves. The temperature of the injectate and the change in temperature in the pulmonary artery are measured by thermistor catheters connected to the computer. The result is presented in litres per minute a few seconds after making the injection, and in one instrument the reading is corrected to the Fick regression line of figure 24.

The advantage of the thermal method is that arterial sampling is unnecessary and measurements may be frequently repeated.

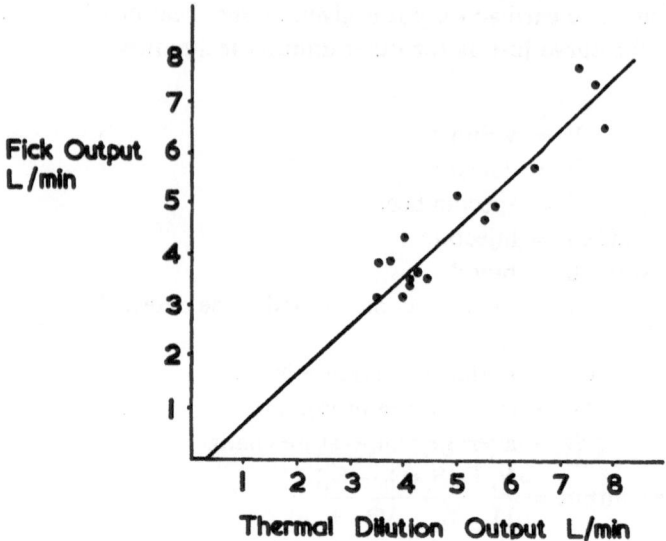

Fig. 24. Correlation between thermal and Fick outputs.

REFERENCES

Bain, W. H. and Harper, A. M., *Blood flow through organs and tissues*. Livingstone, London 1968.

Branthwaite, M. A. and Bradley, R. D., *J. appl. Physiol.* 24, no. 3, 434 (1968).

Chapelle, M. and Mensch, B., *Arch. Maladies du Coeur et des vaisseaux* 62, 1505 (1969).

Clark, C., Ph. D. Thesis, University of London, 1966.

Cross, G. and Light L. H., *J. Phys.* 217, 5 (1971).

Dodge, H. T., Sandler, H., Ballew, D. W. and Lord, J. D., *Amer. Heart J.* 60, 762 (1960).

Feigenbaum, H., *Echocardiography*. Lea & Febiger, Philadelphia 1973.

Feigenbaum, H. Wolfe, S., Popp, R. L., Haine, C. L. and Dodge, H. T., *Amer. J. Cardiol.* 23, 111 (1969).

Gibson, D. G., *Brit. Heart J.* 35, 128 (1973).

Gibson, D. G. and Brown, D., *Proc. roy. Soc. Med.* 67, 140 (1974).

Grayson, J., *J. Physiol.* 118, 54 (1952).

Green, D. C., Carlisle, R., Grant, C. and Bunnell, I., *Circulation* 35, 61 (1967).

Hensel, H., Ruef, J. and Golenhofen, K., *Pflügers Arch. ges. Physiol.* 259, 267 (1961).

Kolin, A., *Proc. Soc. exptl. Biol. Med.* 35, 53 (1936).

Light, L. H., *Nature* 224, 1119 (1969).

Light, L. H., in: *Fluid dynamic measurements in the industrial and medical environments*. Leicester Univ. Press 1972.

Light, L. H., in: *Cardiovascular applications of ultrasound*, ed. R. S. Reneman. North-Holland Pub. Comp., Amsterdam 1974.

Light, L. H. and Cross, G., in: *Blood flow measurement*, ed. C. Roberts. Sector Pub., London 1972.

Marcus, M. L. et al., *Circulation* XLV, 65 (1972).

Mellander, S. and Rushmer, R. F., *Acta Physiol. Scand.* 48, 13 (1960).
Mills, C. J., *Phys. in Med. Biol.* ii, 323 (1966).
Mowbray, J. F., *J. appl. Physiol.* 14, 647 (1959).
Schultz, D. L., Tunstall-Pedoe, D. S., Lee, G. de J., Gunning, A. J. and Bellhouse, B. J.,
    in: *Ciba symposium on circulatory and respiratory mass transport.* J. & A. Churchill,
    London 1969.
Sandler, H. and Dodge, H. T., *Amer. Heart J.* 75, 325 (1968).
Satomura, S. and Kaneko, *3rd Int. Conf. Med. Electronics*, London 1960.
Stegall, H. F., Rushmer, R. F. and Baker, D. W., *J. appl. Physiol.* 21 (2), 707 (1966).

BEAT TO BEAT CARDIAC OUTPUT FROM THE ARTERIAL PRESSURE PULSE CONTOUR

K. H. WESSELING, N. T. SMITH, W. W. NICHOLS, H. WEBER,
B. DE WIT & J. E. W. BENEKEN

INTRODUCTION

Beat-to-beat, or continuous, cardiac output is a measurement that has long been desired for physiological and clinical information. The electromagnetic flow meter (e.m.f.) provides such a measurement. Its prime disadvantage, the necessity of a major operation to place the probe around the ascending aorta, has precluded its use, except for animal experimentation and in occasional cases of open heart surgery. The clinically applicable techniques such as indicator dilution, direct Fick, and X-ray contrast methods only sample the mean cardiac output or stroke volume during selected intervals, widely separated in time. In addition, these techniques require skilled personnel, careful execution, sophisticated equipment, and elaborate calibration procedures. In short, they are difficult measurements from an operational point of view and not well suited for monitoring purposes. On the other hand, blood pressure measurements are relatively simple to obtain, and are continuous and easy to calibrate.

Pressure and flow in arteries are related to each other, as current and voltage or force and displacement are related to each other. This relationship has been explicitly or implicitly used in various forms over a number of years to compute cardiac output from pressure wave form data. These methods were grouped together under the name *pulse contour methods*, and are based on the constant relationship between pressure and flow or pressure and volume changes. Depending on the concept which one has of the arterial system, such as the Windkessel model, or the uniform tube model, different relationships result between pressure and flow or volume.

The major portion of any evaluation of pulse contour methods is proving that the chosen relation is indeed constant, i.e. that the model is correct.

In this paper we will present a new pulse contour method, and a specially designed device (Cardiac Output Computer, COC), which uses this method

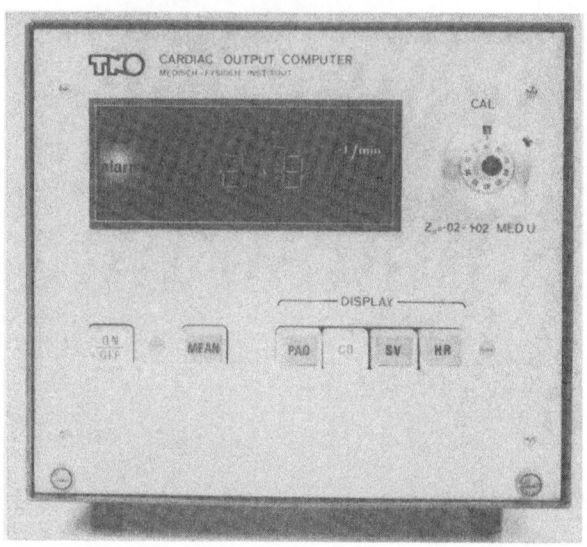

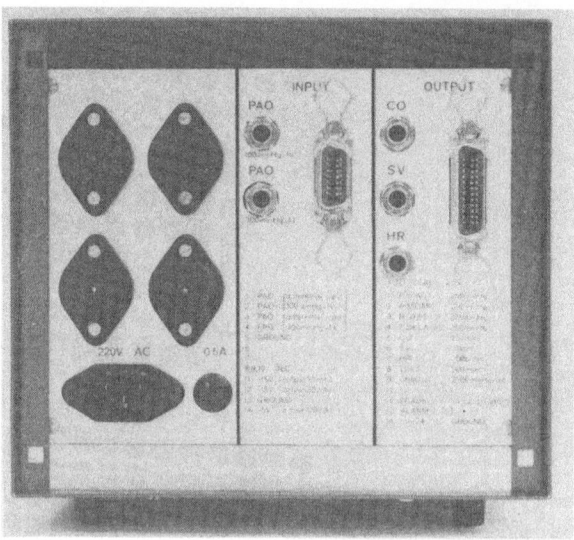

Fig. 1. Photograph of the front and rear panels of the TNO Cardiac Output Computer (COC). The front panel at the top contains the controls and the numerical display. The rear panel below has the input and output connectors and a fuse. The power supply voltage regulators are also mounted on this panel.

to compute beat-to-beat stroke volume, heart rate and cardiac output. Some condensed results of an evaluation in an arterial model, in dog experiments and in human volunteers will be given.

DESCRIPTION OF THE INSTRUMENT

A photograph of the instrument is shown in Fig. 1.

The on/off button and the selection buttons for the display of cardiac output, stroke volume, heart rate or mean arterial pressure are located on the lower part of the front panel. In the upper part is shown the numerical display of the selected quantity together with the appropriate units. An alarm light signals an absent wave form or the presence of distorted pressure wave forms. A patient calibration knob is provided to adjust the displayed values of cardiac output or of stroke volume to match an independent measurement obtained by a standard method. The reason for this single calibration for each patient is explained in subsequent sections.

On the rear panel are located the input and the output connectors. One of two calibrations for the arterial pressure input signal can be selected: 100 mm Hg/V or 300 mm Hg/V, to adapt to the transducer-amplifier output calibration. Output signals are in the form of continuous, calibrated analog voltages, and all signals are present simultaneously. All inputs withstand continuous overloads of up to 250 V and all outputs can be short circuited without affecting the proper operation of the instrument. Triggering is fully automatic and no adjustments need to be made. The internal accuracy of the instrument is $\pm 3\%$. Leakage current of the instrument is 25 μA, with the ground lead interrupted, a level safe for equipment not in direct connection to the patient. Approximate weight of the instrument is 3.5 kg.

METHOD AND APPROXIMATION. USE OF A CONCEPTUAL MODEL

The method used to extract stroke volume information from the pressure contour is illustrated in Fig. 2. The area under the systolic portion of the aortic pressure wave form, divided by a patient constant, Z_0, is equated to left ventricular stroke volume as follows:

$$SV = \frac{1}{Z_0} \int_{syst} \{PAO(t) - PED\} dt.$$

The constant Z_0 is related to the characteristic impedance of the aorta, as explained later. Heart rate is determined as the inverse of the time lapse between two consecutive dicrotic notches. Cardiac output is computed for each beat as the product of stroke volume and heart rate.

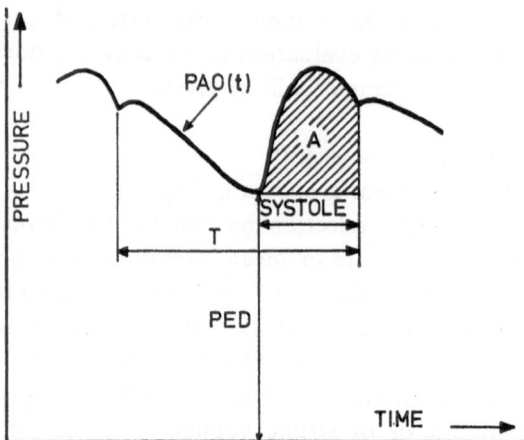

Fig. 2. The method of stroke volume integration is based on computation of the shaded area '*A*' as shown in this figure. Divided by a patient constant Z_0, it delivers the stroke volume. Time lapse T between notches determines the beat-to-beat heart rate. Cardiac output is computed as the product of heart rate and stroke volume,
$$CO = (0.06 \times A)/(T \times Z_0) \ (l/\text{min}).$$

The estimation of stroke volume by this method is based on a conceptual model of the arterial system, but the computations of heart rate and of cardiac output as their product, are straightforward and without further assumptions.

The arterial system in this model is viewed as a uniform, distensible tube with constant cross-sectional area and constant modulus of elasticity along its entire length. Such a tube exhibits the phenomenon of transmission. A pulsatile variation, applied at one end of the tube will propagate along the tube towards the other end and arrive there sometime later. Propagation is accompanied by a temporary change in diameter and pressure. If the diameter change is large the pressure change is also large and the ratio of the change in the diameter squared (the cross-sectional area), to the change in pressure is called the specific compliance of the tube. A change in the diameter and thus of the volume of the tube is not possible without a flow change. The magnitude of the flow depends on the magnitude of the volume change. The ratio of the pressure change to the flow change is determined by the tube's properties and also by the specific density of the fluid that must be accelerated and decelerated in the process and is called characteristic impedance. If the specific density of the filling fluid is known, the characteristic impedance value can be determined from the cross-sectional area and the compliance or distensibility of the tube. It is valid only for pulsatile pressures and flows, unlike the Poisseuille resistance which depends on blood viscosity and the radius of the tube to the fourth power and applies to steady flows and pressures as well as (for small enough diameters) to pulsatile phenomena.

Thus if the tube's characteristic impedance is known, the ratio of pulsatile pressure to pulsatile flow is known, and the pulsatile flow can be computed from a measurement of the pulsatile pressure.

This is the procedure used in the COC.

As there is usually no prior knowledge or direct technique available for determining the value of the characteristic impedance of the aorta of patients, it must be calculated indirectly.

The situation is not as ideal as we have presented it. The aorta is tapered in diameter and the modulus of elasticity is not constant, but increases towards the periphery. In addition, both the aortic diameter and the modulus of elasticity vary with mean pressure. Since the method of stroke volume estimation is based on a constant cross-section and elasticity, it is necessary to investigate the magnitude of error created by these deviations from ideal. Other approximations to the actual physiological situation, such as ignoring the peripheral resistance, are also present, but are of less importance and will not be treated extensively here.

We will first explore the possible changes in the calibration or characteristic impedance (Z_0) with mean distending pressure. Using unpublished curves, assembled by Van der Hoeven of our group, from literature dealing with the radius and radius plus volume changes of human aorta as a function of pressure and age (1, 2), we computed the values of the characteristic impedance. It appears that the radius and consequently the characteristic impedance at a certain pressure level is dependent on age. Three curves are shown in Fig. 3, which gives the value of the characteristic impedance as a function of pressure for age groups of 20, 30 and 50 years. These curves are average curves for a number of subjects. They indicate that the value of characteristic impedance is relatively constant, independent of the actual pressure level for the lowest age group from 40 mm Hg mean pressure upwards, and that there is a moderate increase in the value of Z_0 for the other groups, almost linearly related to the increasing mean pressure level. Correction for this variation could be relatively simple if the mean pressure and the age of the patient are known. The most important conclusion from these curves is that aortic characteristic impedance is a relatively constant,

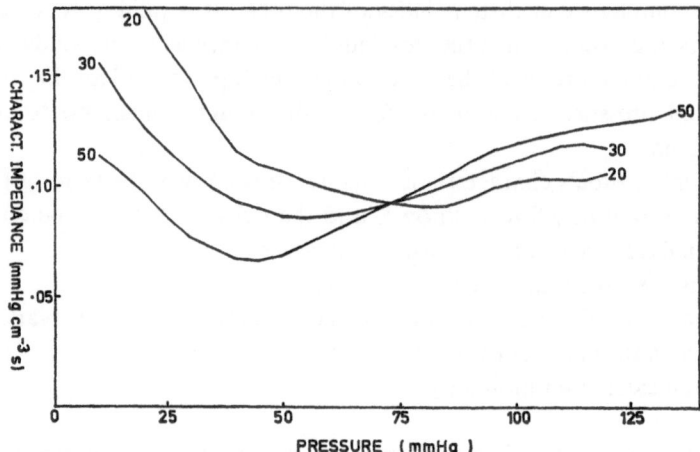

Fig. 3. The value of the characteristic impedance as a function of mean pressure. The characteristic impedance changes somewhat with age. Curves labelled 20, 30 and 50 denote different age groups.

relatively smooth, well behaved, age-dependent function of pressure. Apparently such curves do not preclude the use of this pulse contour method, which is based on the characteristic impedance as a calibration constant as was explained earlier. It should thus be sufficient to determine the actual value of the calibration only once for each patient.

EVALUATION IN AN ANALOG COMPUTER MODEL OF THE HUMAN ARTERIAL SYSTEM

The next factor to be considered is the effect of tapering of the aortic cross-sectional area and accompanying changes in the elastic modulus of the aortic wall. For this purpose we have used an accurate mathematical model of the arterial system which was programmed on an analog computer. The geometry of the model (taper, location of side branches of the aorta, peripheral vascular beds etc.) was taken from the work of De Pater (3). For the programmed visco-elastic properties as a function of position in the model, data from Learoyd and Taylor (4) were taken, adapted for use in computer models, following a procedure and using the results given by Wesseling et al. (5). The resulting model has a realistic, rather strong taper. The model was driven via a valve by a left ventricular pressure wave form generated by a simulator with a variable heart rate (Wesseling et al. (6)). Using the pressure and flow wave forms available in the model, beat-to-beat values of the true stroke volume integrated from the flow pulse and the pulse contour stroke volume from the aortic pressure pulse were computed. Heart rate was varied, and for each setting of heart rate the value of the calibration was adjusted so that for that value of the calibration the true stroke volume and the pulse contour stroke volume were equal. If the pulse contour method is perfect, a constant value for the calibration, independent of heart rate, should result.

In addition to varying heart rate, we programmed the model for three values of total systemic peripheral resistance corresponding to normal, low and high cardiac outputs of 5, 3 and 10 l/min respectively. The calibration should ideally be insensitive to the actual value of the peripheral resistance. Finally, to account for the effects of aortic aging and mean pressure changes on characteristic impedance, models with three different levels of characteristic impedance were programmed corresponding to a normal aorta, a stiff aorta as at old age and high mean arterial pressure, and a compliant aorta as present in young subjects at low mean arterial pressure. A total of nine different models were thus studied (3 values of total peripheral resistance times 3 values of aortic compliance), and heart rate could be varied continuously between 55 and 150 beats per minute.

Fig. 4 illustrates the results. The calibration factor (vertically) is plotted against heart rate (horizontally). Several things are apparent from the curves

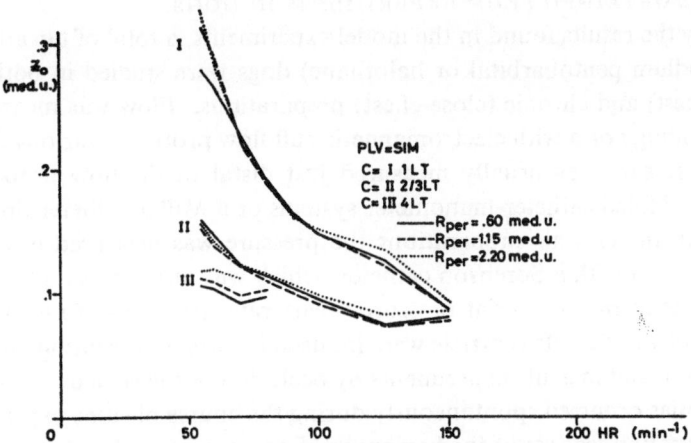

Fig. 4. Values for the calibration factor versus heart rate. Curves are obtained in a mathematical model of the human arterial system, programmed on an analog computer. Each one of the nine curves signifies different model conditions, such as stiff, normal or compliant aortas, or low, normal and high total systemic resistance values.

in this figure. First, the calibration is not independent of heart rate as it ideally should have been. The fact itself can be explained quite simply. The tapering of the aorta means that the characteristic impedance is not a constant, but varies along its length. In fact the value of Z_0 increases gradually from the heart to the periphery. The ratio of pressure change to flow change is thus constantly changing when the ejection pulse from the heart travels towards the periphery. The longer the ejection, the further the pulse travels and the more the increase in impedance it meets on its way. To reiterate, at slow heart rates ejection time is long, the pulse travels further into the aorta and meets higher characteristic impedance values, therefore the calibration Z_0 is higher.

In addition, the variation in the calibration with heart rate is more pronounced for the stiff aorta (curves labelled I) than for the normal (Group II) and again for the compliant aorta (Group III).

The three curves within each of the groups represent different values of total systemic peripheral resistance for the same characteristic impedance level. It is apparent that this pulse contour method is largely independent of the actual value of peripheral resistance.

Again all nine curves are relatively smooth, well behaved functions of heart rate, over the range of heart rates considered, for which variation it should be possible to correct if proved necessary in practice.

RESULTS OBTAINED FROM EXPERIMENTS IN DOGS

To verify the results found in the model experiments, a total of ten anaesthetised (sodium pentobarbital or halothane) dogs were studied in both acute (open-chest) and chronic (close-chest) preparations. Flow was measured in the ascending aorta with electromagnetic cuff flow probes of various designs. Aortic pressure was usually measured just distal to the flow probe using either fluid filled catheter-manometer systems or a Millar catheter tip manometer. In the chronic preparations the pressure was measured in the descending aorta with a Sorenson catheter, which was inserted percutaneously.

Changes in mean arterial pressure, heart rate, peripheral resistance and contractility of the left ventricle were induced by drug intervention and vagal stimulation and in acute experiments by occlusion of the vena cava. Various arrhythmias occurred spontaneously during the course of some experiments. The calibration was set at the beginning of an experiment by comparing the stroke volume integrated from the aortic flow pulse with the stroke volume indicated by the COC from the pressure pulse. After the initial calibration the value of Z_0 was not changed for the remainder of the experiment.

One interesting record is shown in Fig. 5. During the course of this particular open-chest experiment, acute cardiogenic shock occurred. Prior to the segment of the record shown, norepinephrine and ouabaine were administered in order to increase arterial blood pressure and myocardial contractile force and the heart was cooled with ice cubes to decrease the heart rate. During the entire shock and recovery period the computer estimate and the true stroke volume followed each other closely, with differences never greater than 15%. The calibration was unchanged from the 'control' setting at the beginning of the experiment. Evaluation of the results of other interventions lead to the following conclusions valid for dogs.

a) Contrary to the results of the model experiments, changes in heart rate and mean arterial pressure, either individually or simultaneously, did not change the value of the calibration by more than 15% from the original control value. Translated into the concepts used earlier, this could mean that the dog aorta is not as strongly tapered as assumed for the human model (calibration is not strongly dependent on heart rate), and that the curves of characteristic impedance versus mean arterial pressure are essentially flat, similar to those found for young human subjects in Fig. 3.

b) The calibration Z_0 is not significantly dependent on the concentration of sympathomimetic amines in the blood, such as epinephrine and norepinephrine, isoproterenol or metaraminol. This finding differs from the conclusions of Kouchoukos et al. (7) but their conclusions were based on the use of a different pulse contour method.

c) Changes in contractility of the heart, as induced by the administration of $CaCl_2$ or some sympathomimetic amines, do not change the calibration, and the same is true for changes in peripheral resistance. This finding is in accordance with the results from the model experiments.

d) It was also found that this pulse contour method is reliable during various irregular cardiac rhythms, such as bigeminal rhythm, pulsus alternans, atrial fibrillation and premature ventricular contractions, even on a beat-to-beat basis.

e) For the chronic preparations the calibration was constant to within 5% from day to day. This was not found during the acute experiments, where an increase of maximally 35% in the calibration was sometimes noted during the first hour of the operation.

f) Catheters, inserted percutaneously in the femoral artery and positioned in the descending aorta, could be utilized without an apparent reduction in accuracy.

RESULTS OF AN EVALUATION IN YOUNG HEALTHY VOLUNTEER SUBJECTS

A total of 22 experiments were done with 20 volunteer subjects aged 20 to 33 years, who underwent no surgery.

Cardiac output was measured by the dye dilution technique, employing vena caval or right atrial injections of indocyanine green dye and blood withdrawal from a radial arterial catheter. The same catheter was used for the measurement of arterial blood pressure recorded onto an FM magnetic tape recorder. For this evaluation, the *radial arterial pressure* signal was played into the COC and the cardiac output value indicated just before disconnection of the radial catheter, for blood withdrawal through the densitometer, was compared to the subsequently measured dye dilution cardiac output. This non-synchronism in the cardiac output comparisons is a possible source of errors in addition to errors inherent in the particular pulse contour method used. Another such source of error is the use of the radial arterial pressure to replace the aortic pressure wave form as used in the model and animal evaluation.

When radial pressure is utilized, the arm arterial system acts essentially as the catheter, connecting the aorta to the manometer, but that catheter produces a strongly distorted signal wave form. At normal arterial pressure levels, the radial pulse is rounded off and shows oscillations not usually present in the aortic pressure wave form. However, as long as the area under the systolic pulse of the radial artery is the same as that of the aorta, or if there is a constant factor between the two areas, the radial pulse can still be used. In practice, two problems occurred. First, the ratio between the aortic and radial surface areas is clearly not constant. At normal and high mean arterial pressures it is greater than 1 but at low mean arterial pressures it is less than 1, as was verified in model experiments in which these conditions were simulated. Second, the radial pressure pulse at low mean arterial pressures becomes so rounded and smooth, that it was not possible for a human observer or for the COC to find the dicrotic notch, marking the end of ejection. In the following results we have included all situations of low, normal or high mean arterial pressures, as long as the COC was able to recognize a dicrotic notch, although this was frequently located too early in time on smooth, low pressure wave forms. We have not endeavoured to correct for possible errors due to variations in this area ratio. During

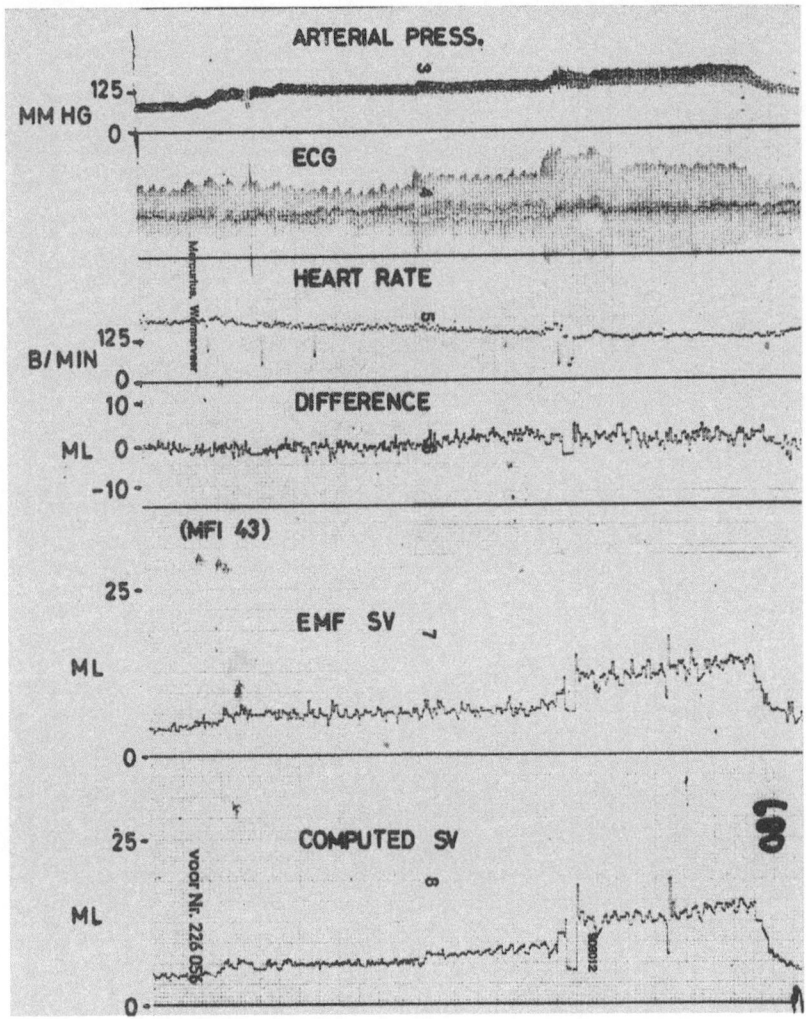

Fig. 5. Recording made during recovery from acute cardiogenic shock in an open-chest, anesthetised dog. Traces signify from above: ascending aortic pressure, ECG, heart rate, the difference between the true stroke volume and the computer estimated stroke volume, the true stroke volume integrated from the ascending aortic cuff flow probe, and the COC-estimated stroke volume from the arterial pressure pulse contour.

each session the hemodynamic conditions of heart rate, peripheral resistance and mean arterial pressure were altered using a variety of pharmacological agents. Usually no more than three of the following agents were administered in any one subject: methoxamine, mephentermine, atropine, halothane, N_2O, fluroxene, isoflurane and hexamethonium (C_6). The calibration was set at the beginning of each session, under control conditions and before the administration of pharmacological agents. A single (usually the first) dye dilution cardiac output was used and compared to the COC output as follows. The calibration was initially set at 0.1. If the dye dilution output reads 5 and the COC output 6.5 l/min, the correct calibration was CAL = $\frac{6.5}{5} \times 0.1 = 0.13$. Regression lines and correlation coefficients were computed for each subject separately, and then averaged over all subjects and the standard deviations computed.

The results are summarized in Table 1, left column.

The mean intercept of the regression line with the y-axis should ideally be zero, but deviates significantly from it. The deviation of the mean slope of the regression line from the ideal value line is also significant. This suggests systematic rather than random errors in the COC method.

Since inspection of the individual curves also suggested the presence of systematic errors with changing heart rate and mean arterial pressure, we attempted to correct these errors, using the curves of characteristic impedance versus mean arterial pressure and those versus heart rate obtained in the model. The corrected results are shown in Table 1, right column. It can be seen that a considerable improvement is obtained. The mean intercept is much closer to the ideal zero value and the standard deviation has decreased. The slope is much closer to one, and its relative standard deviation has decreased by about 30%. The correlation coefficient is closer to one also, with a substantially reduced standard-deviation. The improvement is particularly interesting in view of the fact that model results and literature data used for the correction factor were not connected with the particular experiments evaluated here. This approach is different from that using a theoretically superior multiple regression analysis on the data points to find the correction factors. Some of the remaining errors are ascribed, as mentioned earlier, to the non-synchronous character of the COC-dye dilution cardiac output comparisons, and to the use of the radial artery pressure signal. To our knowledge this is the first time that a pulse contour method has been evaluated using such peripherally recorded pressure signals. It is

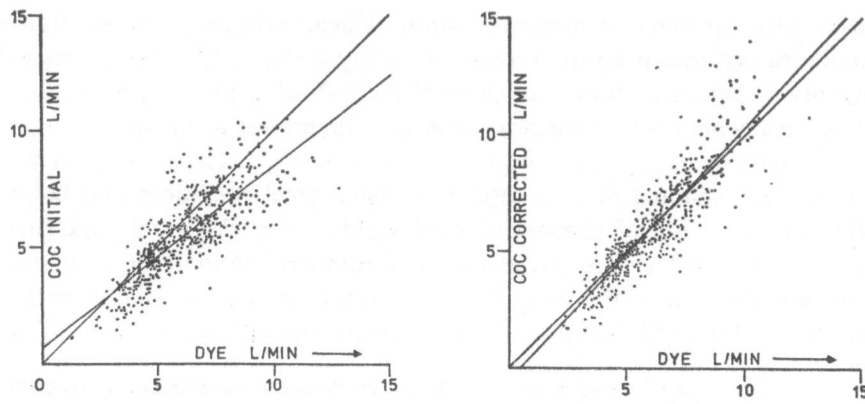

Fig. 6. Comparison of the dye dilution cardiac output with the computer estimated cardiac output, from the pressure pulse contour, obtained in young healthy volunteers. The left plot shows the 'raw data', the right plot after a correction factor has been applied. The COC estimate is plotted vertically from the radial arterial pressure pulse contour, the dye dilution or 'true' cardiac output is plotted horizontally. Regression lines for the 511 comparisons are also shown. The plot and the regression lines include the 22 points used (one for each session) to set the patient calibration Z_0.

clear that the possibility of using such signals widens the range of possible applications of the COC considerably.

Fig. 6 gives the results of all 511 dye dilution-COC comparisons, both for the initial values and for the corrected values. The line of identity 45° line) and the regression line for all points taken together are also shown in this figure. Table 2 lists the values of the regression analysis.

In Fig. 7 the results of two sessions with one volunteer have been plotted, arranged in order of time. The case is particularly interesting because the two sessions were recorded on different days yet, for the corrected COC curves, the calibration value for the first session was also used during the second session more than two months later. The improvement obtained with the correction factor is particularly noteworthy in this case, due to the large variations in mean arterial pressure and especially heart rate. In the first session the effects of methoxamine, and of the sequence atropine-methoxamine were studied. In the second session methoxamine was replaced by mephentermine. Both methoxamine and mephentermine are sympathomimetic amines. Methoxamine raises blood pressure mainly by causing vasoconstriction, mephentermine mainly by cardiac stimulation (8, 9).

In a separate section of Fig. 7 the evaluation of the capacity of the COC

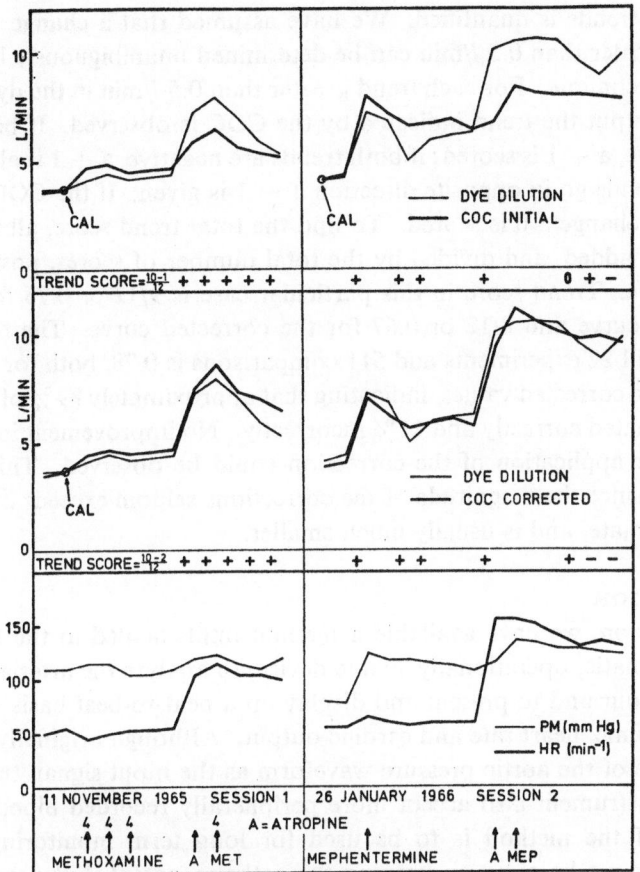

Fig. 7. Plots of the results of a COC-dye dilution comparison in one young healthy volunteer, during two sessions more than two months apart. Measurements are plotted against the number of the comparison. Vertically from above:
a) The reference dye dilution, and the initial COC measurements, and an indication of the trend following capacity for all changes greater than ± 0.5 *l*/min in the dye dilution measurements.
b) The reference dye dilution, and the corrected COC values, (for factors incorporated in the correction factor, see text) and an indication of the trend score. Please note that the calibration of the patient constant as used during the first session on November 11, is also used for the second session on January 26.
c) The heart rate and mean arterial pressure.
d) An indication of the agents used during these two experiments. '*A*' indicates atropine.

to follow trends is quantified. We have assumed that a change in cardiac output greater than 0.5 l/min can be determined unambiguously by the dye dilution technique. For each trend greater than 0.5 l/min in the dye dilution cardiac output the trend indicated by the COC is observed. If both trends are positive, a + 1 is scored; if both trends are negative, a + 1 is also scored. If both trends go in opposite direction a − 1 is given. If the COC estimate shows no change a 0 is scored. To find the total trend score, all individual scores are added, and divided by the total number of scores, positive, zero or negative. Trend score in this particular case is 9/12 or 0.75 for the uncorrected curve and 8/12 or 0.67 for the corrected curve. The total trend score for all 22 experiments and 511 comparisons is 0.78, both for the initial and for the corrected values, indicating that approximately 89 % of all trends were estimated correctly and 11 % incorrectly. No improvement in the trend score after application of the correction could be observed. This is to be expected, since the magnitude of the corrections seldom exceeds 25 % of the initial estimate, and is usually much smaller.

CONCLUSION

In conclusion, we have available a method implemented in the form of a fully automatic, operationally simple device, to analyse the arterial pressure pulse contour and to present and display on a beat-to-beat basis values for stroke volume, heart rate and cardiac output. Although originally designed for the use of the aortic pressure waveform as the input signal, the method and the instrument also accept more peripherally recorded blood pressure signals. If the method is to be used for long term monitoring, special attention must be given to keeping the catheter patent, but commercially available continuous flush attachments have usually been adequate.

Evaluations of the method and the instrument in dogs and in young healthy volunteers suggest a clinically useful accuracy over a wide range of hemodynamic conditions. A correction factor, which includes mean arterial pressure and heart rate must be applied to the human results. For dogs this correction does not appear to be necessary.

An initial calibration is necessary for each patient separately. For this a clinical estimate of cardiac output can be used or an absolute measurement of stroke volume or cardiac output by some other means. The calibration appears to be essentially constant over periods of at least several months, in both dog and man.

Table 1.

Averaged results of a regression analysis, executed for each experiment separately, for a total of 22 experiments with 20 young healthy volunteers (mean $\pm$ 1 standard deviation). The regression equation was $y = a + bx$, in which y is the COC estimate of cardiac output, taken 1 or 2 minutes before the dye dilution cardiac output x. The column 'initial' represents the original COC estimates of cardiac output, the 'corrected' column gives COC estimates corrected for the systematic errors introduced by changes in mean pressure and heart rate, using a correction factor derived from an analog computer model.

The maximum and minimum values for cardiac output, mean pressure and heart rate observed in the experiments are also given.

	Initial		*Corrected*
number of comparisons per experiment	23 ± 10		23 ± 10
intercept a [*l*/min]	1.67 ± 1.95		-0.41 ± 1.45
slope b	0.67 ± 0.24		1.07 ± 0.28
correlation coefficient	0.76 ± 0.18		0.88 ± 0.08
cardiac output range (dye dilution) [*l*/min]	1.3	—	13
mean pressure range [mmHg]	45	—	145
heart rate range [beats/min]	40	—	165

Table 2.

Results of a regression analysis on the pooled data from 22 experiments with 20 young healthy volunteers. 'Initial' and 'Corrected' values are as defined earlier for table 1.

	Initial	*Corrected*
total number of comparisons	511	511
intercept [*l*/min]	0.70	-0.55
slope	0.78	1.08
correlation coefficient	0.81	0.89

REFERENCES

1. Wagner, R. & Kapal E., Ueber Eigenschaften des Aorten Windkessels. *Z. Biol.* 105, 283 (1952).
2. Bader, H., Dependence of wall stress in the human thoracic aorta on age and pressure. *Circ. Res.* 20, 354 (1967).
3. Pater, L. de, *An electrical analogue of the human circulatory system.* Groningen 1966.
4. Learoyd, B. M. & Taylor, M. G., Alterations with age in the visco-elastic properties of human arterials walls. *Circ. Res.* 18, 278 (1966).
5. Wesseling, K. H., Weber, J. A. P. & Wit, B. de, Estimated five component visco-elastic model parameters for human arterial walls. *J. Biomechanics* 6, 13 (1973).
6. Wesseling, K. H., Weber, J. A. P. & Wit, B. de, Variable heart rate electronic simulator for some haemodynamic signals. *Med. & Biol. Engng.* 11, 214 (1973).
7. Kouchoukos, N. T., Sheppard, L. C. & McDonald, D. A., Estimation of stroke volume in the dog by a pulse contour method. *Circ. Res.* 26, 611 (1970).
8. Innes, I. R. & Nickerson, M., Sympathomimetic drugs (chapter 24). In: Goodman, L. S. & Gilman, A. (eds.), *The pharmacological basis of therapeutics,* New York 1968.
9. Smith, N. T., Pressor agents. *Calif. Med.* 107, 33 (1967).

PLETHYSMOGRAPHY IN CLINICAL MEASUREMENT

J. C. DORLAS

When preparing a paper for a Boerhaave course one is involuntarily reminded of Boerhaave's outstanding personality and talents. His scientific capacities in the field of botany and chemistry have worldwide fame and his part in the development of medicine has given him a place in history. Like Sylvius before him he propagated the method of clinical medicine. His clinical bedside teaching has remained the base of medical education until the present day (1).

At Groningen we may be considered faithful disciples of Boerhaave because we still rely largely on clinical observation both at the bedside and in the operating room. In anaesthesia we have to watch all the vital functions of the patient, but for the moment I shall confine myself to only one of these vital functions, namely the circulation.

In circulatory care nowadays, less emphasis is placed on given arterial blood pressure and far more on tissue perfusion. Clinical parameters that give sensitive and early warning against declining tissue perfusion were given several years ago by Lillehei (2). They are summarized in the following table

Table 1. Clinical parameters of the circulation.

SYMPTOM	AS AN INDEX OF
Pulse pressure	Cardiac output
Temperature, color and humidity of the skin at the extremities	State of contraction of the peripheral vessels
Peripheral venous filling	Effective circulating volume
Central venous pressure	Capacity of the heart to cope with the offered venous return
Urine production	Perfusion of the visceral organs.

(Table 1) and are still hold true. Of these parameters, frequent observation of the skin at the extremities is a typical bedside method. To those who are trained and experienced in this respect it gives useful and early practical information (3).

However, to sail by watchful observation alone doesn't give exact data, nor can they be used for scientific purposes. In order to obtain more objective data, plethysmography offers many possibilities. It may be used in several ways to study different aspects of the circulation. To measure blood flow at the level of the fingers, digital plethysmography is a recognized method.

Foster Neumann and Rovenstine (4) reported on pneumoplethysmography to measure digital blood flow.

Schneiderman (5), refering to Foster's work, made use of piezo-electric-crystal plethysmography.

By calculating the area under the digital pulse wave an estimation of the peripheral pulsatile blood flow is accomplished (Fig. 1). The resultant

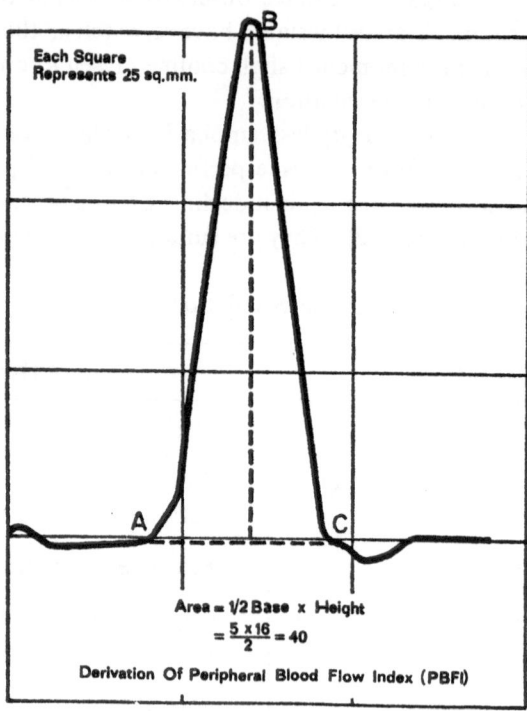

Fig. 1. Calculation of the area under the digital pulse wave (Schneiderman).

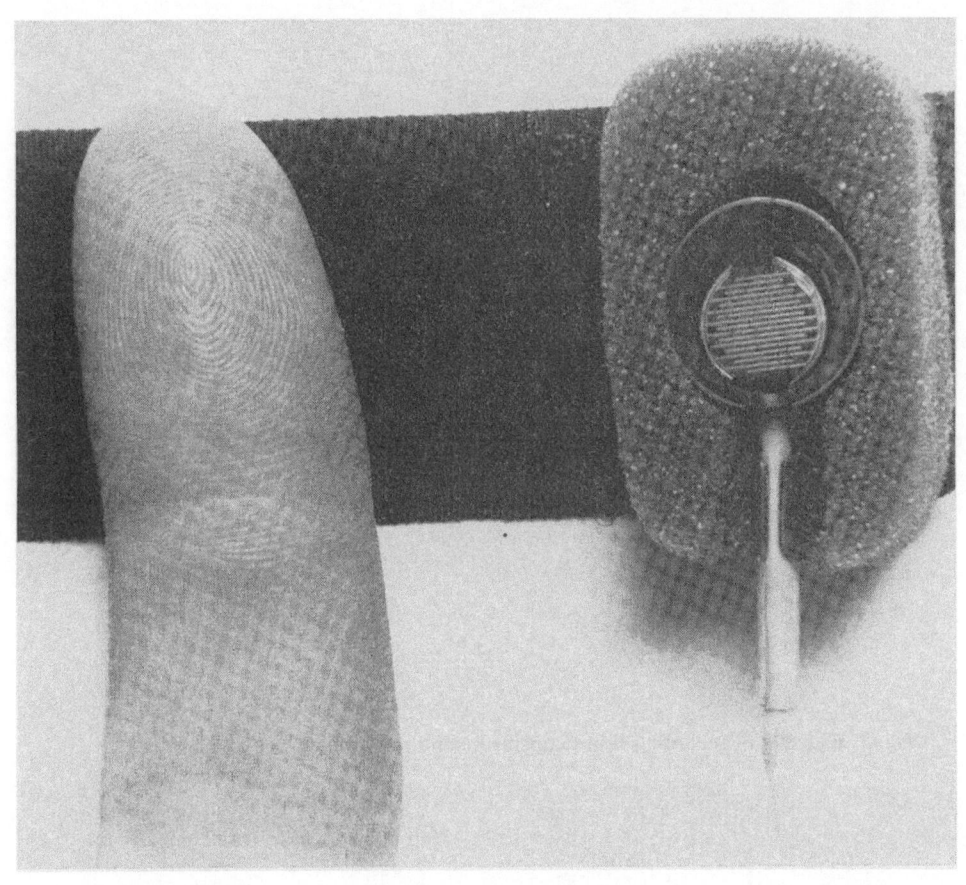

Fig. 2. Digital photosensitive pulse detector.

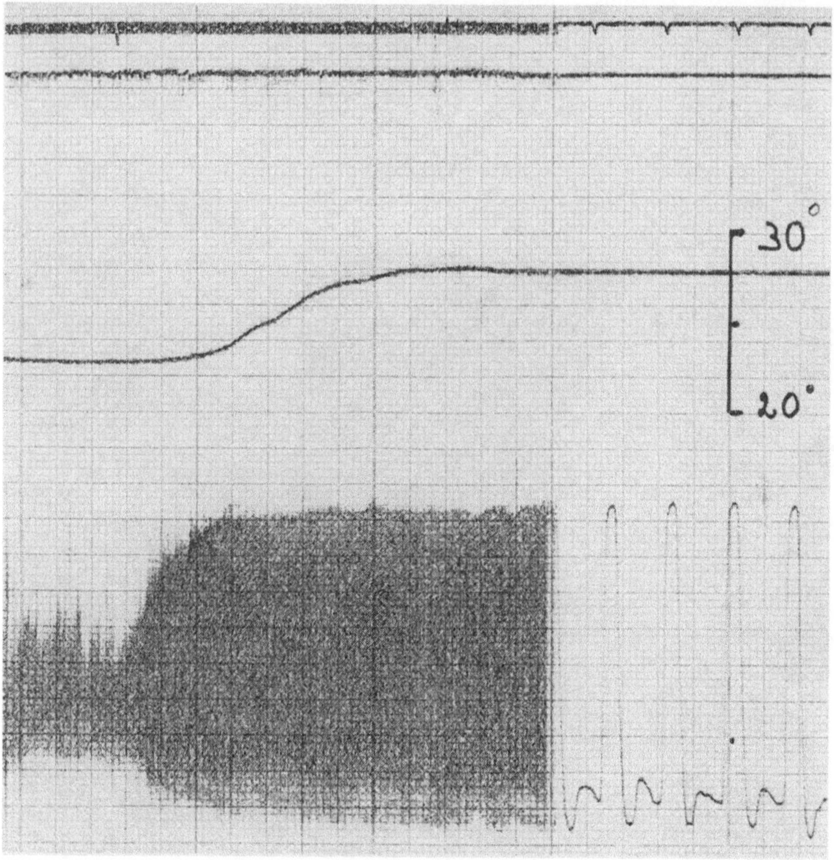

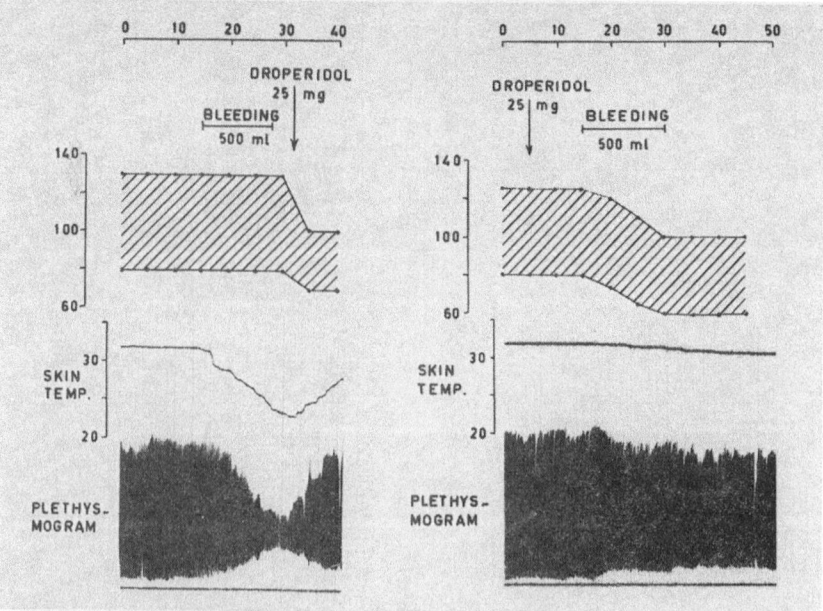

Fig. 3. Example of recording skin temperature and plethysmogram simultaneously.

Fig. 4. Different reactions of the circulation to bleeding.

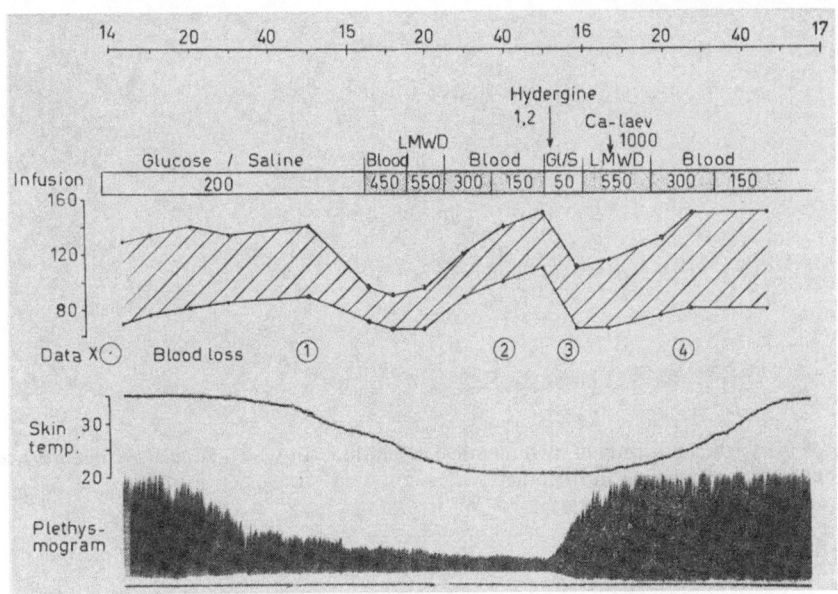

Fig. 5. Circulatory changes due to serious blood loss and its treatment.

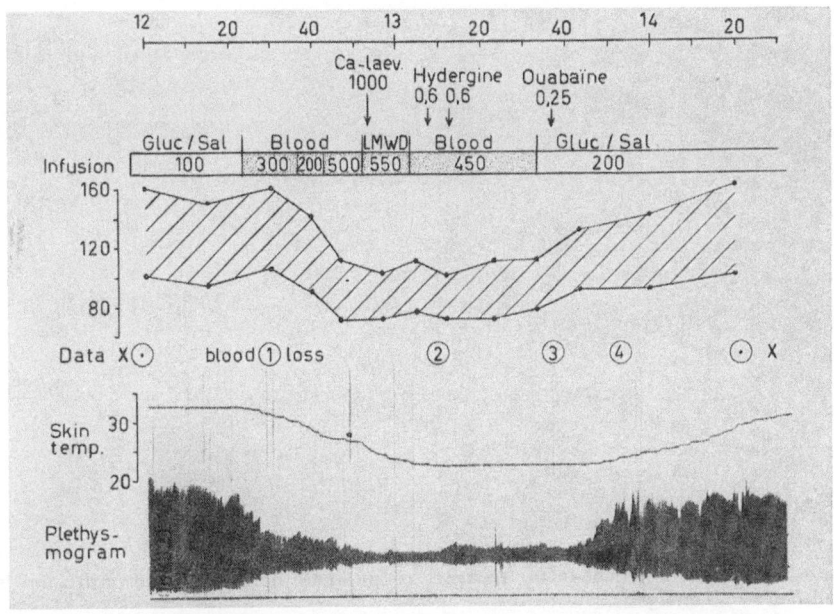

Fig. 6. Haemodynamic disturbance in which a cardiac cause seems responsible.

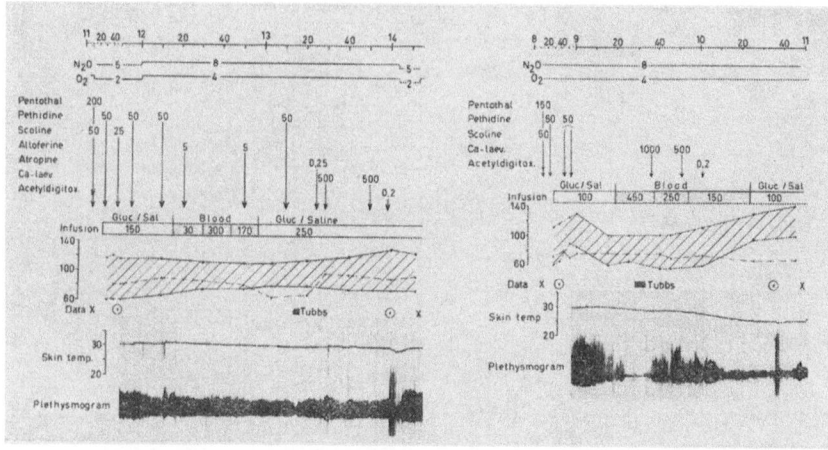

Fig. 7. Anaesthetic records of two identical operations in which circulatory disturbance in one is far greater than in the other.

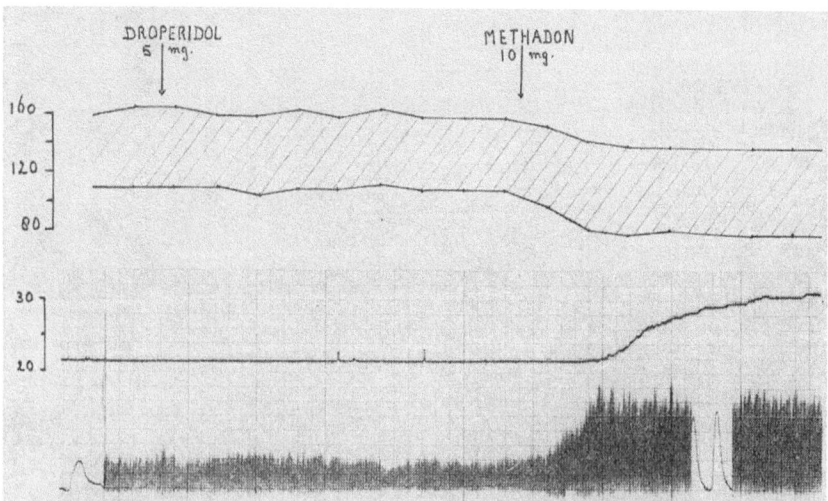

Fig. 8. Records of a patient in the recovery room where peripheral vasoconstriction is abolished by an analgesic.

'Peripheral Blood Flow Index' may be compared with the indexes calculated at any other moment.

Mercury-in-rubber strain gauges are used to measure forearm and calf blood flow simultaneously by Payne and his collaborators (6). The analogue outputs from these transducers are transmitted to a computer. The blood flows are calculated on-line.

Johnstone (7), however, states that forearm plethysmography cannot be interpreted accurately because the response to sympathetic stimulation of the vessels in this area is of two kinds, i.e. a mixture of dilatation of the vessels of the skeletal muscles, which are beta-receptoractivated, and constriction of the vessels of the skin and subcutaneous tissue. This shows that detailed interpretation of plethysmography is still open to discussion. Therefore we have avoided going into this controversial matter and have only paid attention to changes in amplitude.

For our simple method of photoplethysmography the detector was initially constructed in 1961 by our Department of Medical Physics (8, 9). A small built-in lamp emits light which enters the skin and is absorbed, reflected and scattered (Fig. 2). The returning light is detected by a photosensitive resistance (Light Dependant Resistance) placed in the centre of the probe. The intensity of the light returning to the detector depends primarily on the properties of the skin. The variations are due to fluctuations in the amount of blood in the finger, i.e. indirectly to the bloodflow. The output signal is recorded graphically.

We combine plethysmography with measurement of skin temperature on the patient's finger or toe. Both phenomena are recorded simultaneously on very slow moving paper (9 cm/hour). The different parts are assembled on a mobile cart.

Fig. 3 shows an example of these recordings. The curve for the skin temperature gives more or less absolute values, but the plethysmogram only gives relative results, so that only changes in amplitude can be demonstrated.

The changes which occur when 500 ml's of blood are taken from a healthy volunteer are shown in Fig. 4. In the left figure we see that the blood pressure remains remarkably constant during this period. This is obviously due to compensatory vasoconstriction. This is confirmed by a fall in the skin temperature and a decrease in the amplitude of the plethysmogram. These changes are reversed if a vasodilator, such as dehydrobenzperidol, is injected intravenously. Only then does the blood pressure fall.

The righthand figure shows what happens when the vasodilator is injected 15 min before the blood is taken. Now the bleeding and the fall in blood

pressure occur simultaneously and the peripheral circulation is little influenced.

Fig. 5 gives the anaesthetic record of a patient with multiple fractures,
entailing rapid and heavy blood loss.

The changes in the skin temperature and plethysmogram indicate a reduction in peripheral perfusion and this occurs long before the drop in arterial
blood pressure (1). Obviously the lost volume should have been replaced
at an earlier stage. Rapid transfusion produces a rise in the bloodpressure
(2), but the decreased peripheral perfusion remains unaltered. This improves
markedly after a vasodilator (1.2 mg of Hydergine) is given (3). The blood
pressure which drops concurrently is restored by means of further transfusion.

Besides hypovolaemia haemodynamic disturbances can also be produced
by a low cardiac output. The anaesthetic record of a patient of 67 years
with a fractured neck of femur illustrates such a state of affairs and is shown
in Fig. 6.

Blood loss certainly plays some part in producing the changes, but
restoring lost volume (1) does not produce an increase in peripheral perfusion
nor in blood pressure. On the contrary a rise in central venous pressure
occurs, although this is not shown in the record.

Since the possibility of overtransfusion is considered 1.2 mg of Hydergine
is injected (2), but produces no improvement: peripheral perfusion remains
low and central venous pressure high. A cardiac cause now seems obvious
and the giving of 1/4 mg of Strophantine (3) indeed produces the desired
effect, i.e. a rise in blood pressure, an increase in the amplitude of the
plethysmogram and a rise in skin temperature.

In Fig. 7 are shown the records of two patients with mitral stenosis who
underwent Tubb's commissurotomies. For the patient on the right it was
the first operation, for the other it was the third, i.e. second relapse. Both
patients were anaesthetised with a barbiturate nitrous oxide/oxygen and
pethidine.

Judging from the course of the two blood pressure curves both anaesthetics
went smoothly, but comparison of the two plethysmograms shows that
circulatory disturbance in one was far greater than that in the other. These
objective data correspond well with the clinical impression of the anaesthetist who was not aware of what was on the records.

The records of a patient treated postoperatively in the recovery room are
given in Fig. 8. Clinical observation showed all the signs of severe peripheral
vasoconstriction (cold and cyanotic hands, nails and lips, empty peripheral
veins, etc.). To combat this, dehydrobenzperidol was given but had little

or no effect. The giving of an analgesic, however, produced considerable clinical improvement as the extremities became warm and pink with prominent veins. These bedside findings correspond very well with the recorded data shown in the figure.

In all these examples distinct disturbances in peripheral perfusion are demonstrated. In anaesthetic practice these changes are generally assessed by watchful observation. However, this needs some training and experience, so that for educational purposes a more objective method is needed.

Also for research purposes we must be able to compare different clinical situations by objective means. The purpose of this paper is to show that even a simple method of clinical measurement can be very adequate in this respect.

REFERENCES

1. Lindeboom, G. A., *Herman Boerhaave, The man and his work.* Butler and Tanner, London 1968.
2. Lillehei, R. C., Dietzman, R. H. & Block, J. H., In: *Cardiac surgery,* Norman, J. C., Butterworths, London 1967.
3. Dorlas, J. C., Bartstra, M. & Zeelenberg, H. J., The use of different drugs in circulatory care during anaesthesia. *Ars Medici, l'Anesthésie vigile et subvigile.* Travaux du sumposium international d'Ostende, Vol. I, Tome III-107 Juin 1970.
4. Foster, A. D., Neumann, C. & Rovenstine, E. A., Peripheral circulation during anaesthesia, shock and hemorrhage. The digital plethysmograph as a clinical guide. *Anaesthesiology* 6, 246 (1945).
5. Schneiderman, B. I., Qualitative measurement of digital blood flow during fluothane anaesthesia. *Proceedings of the second Europ. Congress of Anesthesiology* I, 649, Copenhagen 1966.
6. Payne, J. P., Personal communication (1972).
7. Johnstone, M., The cardiovascular effects of oxytocic drugs. *Brit. J. Anaesth.* 44, 826 (1972).
8. Pater, L. de, Berg, Jw. van den & Buene, A. A., A very sensitive photoplethysmograph using scattered light and a photosensitive resistance. *Acta Physiol. Pharmacol. Neerlandica* 10, 378-390 (1962).
9. Berg, Jw. van den & Vafi, A., A very sensitive two channel photoplethysmograph, the vasotest for peripheral vascular surgery. *Proceedings Kon. Ned. Academie van Wetenschappen,* Series C, 66 no 1, 30-36 (1963).

MEASUREMENT OF CEREBRAL PERFUSION

M. S. CHRISTENSEN

IDEAL CBF TECHNIQUE

An ideal technique should be non-invasive, i.e. neither arterial nor veni-puncture should be necessary. Unfortunately the most informative CBF techniques of today all include cannulation of the internal carotid artery. Furthermore an ideal technique should provide instantaneous and repeatable flow values, e.g. monitoring of moment to moment changes of the flow should be possible. Unfortunately, todays techniques require at least two minutes of steady state conditions to obtain a single flow value, and at least 15 minutes before a repitition will provide comparable flow values.

An ideal technique should measure not only the total flow of the cerebral hemisphere, but also the flow in various regions of the hemisphere. This demand may be fulfilled today, where the flow in up to 256 small regions of a hemisphere may be measured simultaneously, but the problem of iden-tifying non-perfused regions is not solved.

In addition to flow, the substrate metabolism both globally and regionally should be measured. Quite recently a technique meeting this demand has been under development.

The first relevant cerebral perfusion studies in man were described by Lennox and Gibbs in 1932 (1). They measured the cerebral arteriovenous oxygen difference $((A-V)O_2)$ and proposed a parallel relationship to the speed of blood flow: decrease of $(A-V)O_2$ indicates a flow increase and vice versa. The figures obtained were related to flow but not absolute flow rate. The primary assumption to justify the method was a constant cerebral metabolic rate of oxygen $(CMRO_2)$ from study to study. On the other hand this technique may provide instantaneous and repeatable flow values.

The real epoch-making contribution to clinical CBF measurements was made by Kety and Schmidt in 1945 (2) when they first described the classical nitrous oxide method for quantitative determination of CBF in unaneasthe-tized man. Since then several modifications and more and more advanced

CBF techniques had been evaluated, all based on the use of *inert gas clearance*. Some of these methods will de described in detail below.

OUTFLOW DETECTION
Kety – Schmidt technique:
The technique is based on the *principle of Fick* which states that the blood flow through an organ equals the product of the uptake of an inert tracer in the organ, and the concentration difference of the inert tracer between the arterial and venous side of the organ. If the brain is perfused with a diffusible inert gas, it will be taken up by the tissue until it is in equilibrium with the blood concentration of the gas, i.e. tissue concentration = blood concentration x tissue/blood partition coefficient of the inert gas. The gas has to be inert to avoid biochemical reactions or pharmacological actions. Kety and Schmidt used 15 per cent nitrous oxide as the inert gas. It was inhaled for a period of 10 or 15 minutes during which several simultaneous blood samples were drawn from an artery and the jugular bulb for determination of nitrous oxide concentration. When equilibration was completed the nitrous oxide uptake in the ipsilateral hemisphere could be expressed as jugular bulb concentration times brain/blood partition coefficient of nitrous oxide. The mean cerebral arteriovenous nitrous oxide difference during the equilibration period could be derived mathematically from the arterial and cerebral venous concentration curves obtained during the saturation period.

Studying young men at rest Kety and Schmidt (3) found when a 10 minutes equilibration period was used, an average CBF_{10}: 54 (SD $\pm$ 12)ml (blood)/100 g (brain)/min. Furthermore the average cerebral $(A-V)O_2$ was: 6.3 (SD $\pm$ 1.2) volume per cent. $CMRO_2$ was calculated as CBF $\times$ $(A-V)O_2$ giving an average value of: 3.3 (SD $\pm$ 0.4)ml(O_2)/100 g (brain)/min. The cerebral vascular resistance (CVR) was calculated as the ratio between mean arterial blood pressure (MABP) and CBF giving an average value of 1.6 (SD $\pm$ 0.4) in these young men.

Valid flow data with inhalation technique is only obtained when the inspiratory concentration of the tracer is constant during the equilibration period. Another important source of error is the assumption that jugular bulb blood is representative of the venous outflow of the hemisphere. Because contamination with venous blood from extracranial tissues may occur, depending on the jugular sampling technique used.

The clinical application of the method implies the inherent risks of arterial and jugular bulb cannulation. Steady state conditions ($PaCO_2$ and MABP) of at least 10 to 15 minutes are mandatory. As the flow figures are average values of the hemisphere, regions with low or zero perfusion will not be suspected. On the other hand the method gives the opportunity for a simultaneous study of cerebral metabolic parameters. The validity of the equation stating that the rate of tissue metabolism (uptake or release) equals blood flow times arteriovenous concentration difference of the metabolite, has been analyzed by Zierler (4). He depicted the limitations caused by non-steady states: (a) flow variations with time, (b) uptake or output variations with time, and (c) variation of arterial concentration with time.

Modification of Kety – Schmidt technique:

In 1955 Lassen and Munck (5) introduced the use of a radioactive tracer instead of nitrous oxide. They used inhalation of the isotope 85 Kr and counted the beta activity present in the blood samples with a Geiger – Müller tube. An example of a CBF study with this method is shown in Fig. 1. The (ideal or true) flow is calculated according to the equation:

$$CBF_\infty = \lambda \times H/A \times 100 \qquad (1)$$

where λ is the brain/blood partition coefficient of 85 Kr, H is the height of the blood concentration when followed to infinity, and A is the area between the arterial and venous curves when followed to infinity. But for practical purposes and by convention a period of 10 minutes is normally used (cfr. 15 minutes in Fig. 1):

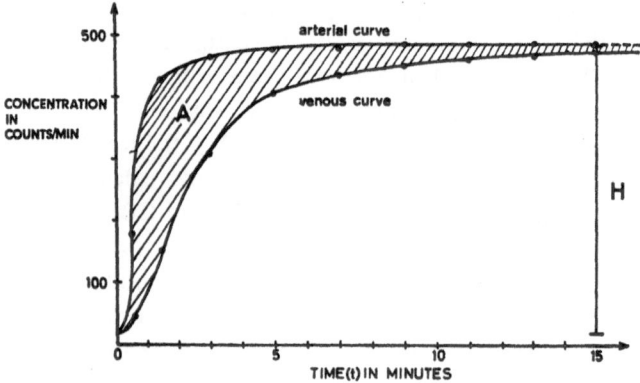

Fig. 1. CBF study using a modification of the Kety–Schmidt technique (radioactive isotope as tracer). The multiple arterial and jugular bulb tracer concentrations are plotted against time. For calculation of CBF_{15}, A_{15} (shaded area until 15 minutes between arterial and venous curves) and H_{15} (height of arterial curve at 15 minutes subtracted background activity) are used.

$$CBF_{10} = \lambda \times H_{10}/A_{10} \times 100 \qquad (2)$$

where A_{10} is the area between the curves when followed 10 minutes only. Compared to the true flow, this calculation will give an overestimation of approximately 10 per cent, because the tail part of the curves are omitted. The normal values found by Lassen and Munck (5) were in agreement with the original values listed above.

RESIDUE DETECTION
Intra-arterial injection technique:
A new approach to CBF measurements using inert gas clearance was described by Lassen and Ingvar in 1961 (6) and by Ingvar and Lassen in 1962 (7). After injection of an isotope dissolved in saline as a 'slug' into a cerebral artery, one observes what is essentially a single transit of a tracer bolus. In the beginning the common carotid artery was used for injection of 85 Kr and the beta activity was followed on the exposed brain surface because of the low penetration ability of beta emission. However, measuring the gamma-emission by a scintillation counter allows extracranial detection of the clearance rate of isotope from brain tissue (8). As the isotope 133 Xe has a higher gamma emission, this has become the tracer of choice.

An extracranially recorded isotope clearance curve is illustrated in Fig. 2. According to Zierler (9), the CBF may be calculated using equation (1) and (2). As mentioned above, the approximation CBF_{10} is an overestimation (about 15 per cent) of the true flow, as A_{10} excludes the tail part of the

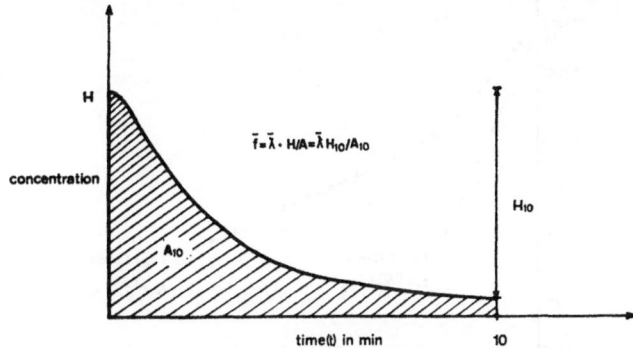

Fig. 2. CBF study using intra-arterial injection of radioactive isotope and extracranial recording of the clearance. The residue activity is plotted against time. For calculation of CBF_{10}, A_{10} (shaded area below clearance curve followed until 10 minutes) and H_{10} (difference between initial height and height at 10 minutes, both corrected for background activity) are used.

clearance curve, when followed to infinity. This stochastic analysis of the clearance curve is often named the *'height over area method'*. Lassen and Høedt Rasmussen (10) have made a comparison of the Kety – Schmidt method (tissue saturation with detection of tracer leaving the organ) and the intra-arterial injection method (detection of residue tracer inside the tissue). They found a close relation between the two methods both theoretically and experimentally.

One of the main sources of error is recirculation of the tracer injected. Small amounts of the indicator gas remain in the pulmonary capillary blood after equilibrium with alveolar air. For correction of CBF the degree of recirculation may be evaluated by a small intravenous injection of the same amount of tracer and recording of the cerebral clearance (11). The recirculation will increase when lung pathology with pulmonary shunting is present. Furthermore correction should be made for remaining radio-activity from a previous study.

Modification for two-compartmental analysis:
By injection of the isotope in the internal carotid artery the clearance curve will only record brain tissue without any extracranial contamination. If the recorded clearance curve is plotted on a logarithmic y - axis against time, it will be a seemingly mono-exponential curve after about five to seven minutes with a half-time (T $\frac{1}{2}$) of the order of five minutes (Fig. 3). Per-

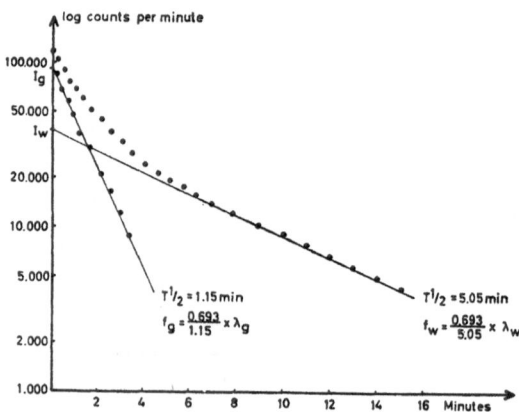

Fig. 3. Two-compartmental analysis ('exponential stripping') of a clearance curve plotted on a logarithmic y-axis against time. The slow component (T $\frac{1}{2}$ = 5.05 min) is subtracted from the composite clearance curve giving the fast component (T $\frac{1}{2}$ = 1.15 min). The zero time intercepts of the slow and fast component curves are I_w and I_g respectively.

forming 'exponential stripping' of the clearance curve, i.e. by subtracting the described mono-exponential curve from the composite clearance curve, a second mono-exponential curve is obtained with a T $\frac{1}{2}$ of the order of one minute. Referring to the two-compartments-in-parallel model, the fast clearance component represents cerebral gray matter (g) and the slow one white matter (w).

According to Hoedt–Rasmussen and coworkers (11) the CBF calculations are made using the equations:

$$CBF_g = \lambda_g \times \frac{0.693}{T\frac{1}{2}_g} \times 100 \tag{3}$$

and

$$CBF_w = \lambda_w \times \frac{0.693}{T\frac{1}{2}_w} \times 100 \tag{4}$$

where λ is the brain/blood partition coefficient of 133 Xe (varies with the hemoglobin concentration). Hoedt–Rasmussen and coworkers (11) had furthermore shown that an estimation of the relative weights of gray (Wg) and white (Ww) matter may be obtained using the equations:

$$W_g = (I_g/CBF_g)/(I_g/CBF_g + I_w/CBF_w) \tag{5}$$

and

$$W_w = (1 - W_g) \tag{6}$$

where I_g and I_w are the zero time intercepts of the fast and slow curve component respectively (Fig. 3).
The normal values obtained are: $CBF_g = 80$ ml/100 g/min; $CBF_w = 20$ ml/100 g/min and $W_g/W_w = 1$.

Modification for initial slope analysis:
By the use of several scintillation detectors and an appropriate collimation it should be possible to make flow measurements in small circumscribed areas of the brain (12, 13). But regional probes show considerable overlapping caused by various factors: (a) by reducing the area scanned by the counter one reduces the number of emissions reaching the counter, (b) gamma emission produces Compton scatter (secondary emission from within the area) which will be registered, (c) 133 Xe undergoes considerable self-absorption in the brain. The counting geometry of a multiple channel detector system is shown in Fig. 4.

The basic idea of initital slope analysis is that the gray matter dominates the initial one to two minutes of the clearance curve, so that it may be regarded as mono-exponential. Analyzing the clearance curve of the first

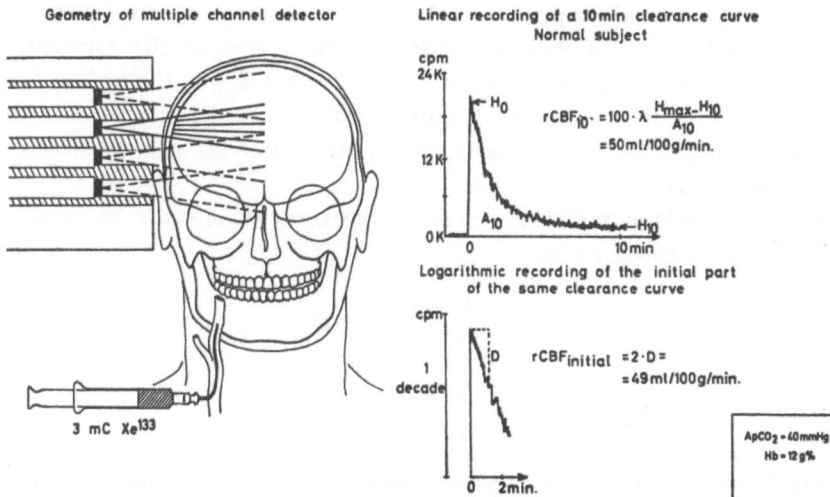

Fig. 4. In the left half of the figure the counting geometry of the multiple scintillation detector system is shown. At the right upper part a stochastic analysis of the clearance curve from a single scintillation detector is shown. At the right lower part an initial slope analysis of the same clearance curve is shown.

minute alone (logarithmically displayed) gives the equation for CBF calculation:

$$CBF_{initial} = 2 \times D_{initial} \times 100 \qquad (7)$$

where 2 is the product of 2,30 (factor for converting base 10 to natural logarithm) and 0,87 (λ_g), and $D_{initial}$ is the numerical value of the initial slope of the clearance curve in base 10 logarithmic system (in fraction of decade per minute; see Fig. 4). As normal value of $CBF_{initial}$ Olesen and co-workers (13) found: 64 (SD $\pm$ 9) ml/100 g/min. Because the $CBF_{initial}$ does not reveal anything about the slow flow components, $CBF_{second\ minute}$ has been suggested as a semi-quantitative measure (calculated using the slope of the second minute of the clearance curve). A two-minute flow index has also been suggested, but the calculations are complicated and the necessary mono-exponential fit of that part of the curve is too uncertain.

Correction for remaining activity from previous measurements is somewhat difficult when initial slope analysis is used. To reduce the problem a sufficiently long time-interval between measurements has to be used (at least 15 minutes).

Olesen and coworkers (13) have compared the values obtained by the different CBF techniques. $CBF_{initial}$ was found to be 20 to 30 per cent lower than CBF_g. A linear relationship was found between $CBF_{initial}$ and CBF_{10} when CBF_{10} was higher than 20 ml/100 g/min. Furthermore W_g estimates are not justified (without anatomical correlation) when CBF_∞ is not above 30 ml/100 g/min.

For clinical use a 35 channel recording system based on the initial slope analysis has been evaluated at Bispebjerg Hospital. The 35 clearance curves are displayed logarithmically during the first two minutes on an oscilloscope screen and photographed with a Polaroid camera (Fig. 5). The method only demands a steady state condition of two minutes but, because of remaining radioactivity, flow measurements may be repeated at 15-minute intervals only. The negatives from the Polaroid camera are transparent and this makes a rapid semiquantitative evaluation possible by superimposing the negatives from two subsequent measurements. By a simple mechanical arrangement the slope of the clearance curve of the first minute can be direct-ly read out as $CBF_{initial}$. The method is especially suitable for the deter-mination of inter-regional differences in flow, and for the study of flow changes within a single patient.

A further refinement of the regional flow technique has been reported by

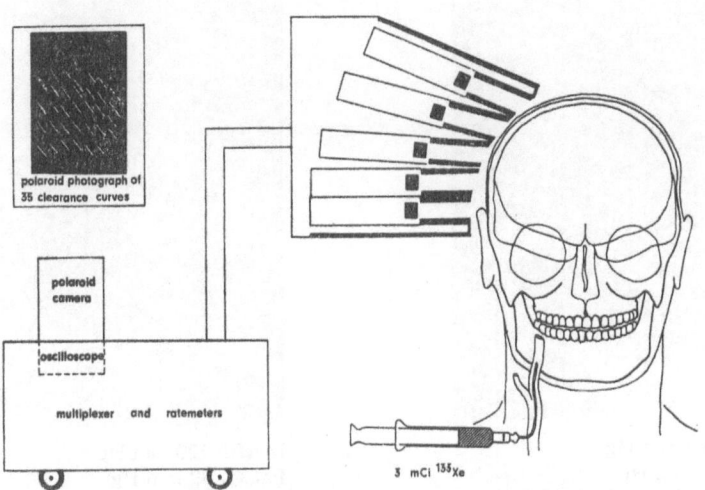

Fig. 5. A 35 channel recording arrangement used at Bispebjerg Hospital in Copenhagen. Pulses from each collimated scintillation detector are displayed logarithmically on an oscilloscope screen via a separate ratemeter and a multiplexer, and photographed with a Polaroid camera during the first two minutes after intra-arterial (internal carotid) injection of 133 Xe.

Sveinsdottir and Lassen (14). They used a dynamic gamma camera based on 256 scintillation crystals. Coupled on-line to a small computer, the results – depicted in analog manner using a color scale or a gray tone scale – were obtained with practically no delay on an oscilloscope and on a colour TV.

TEST OF VASOMOTOR FUNCTION

CBF values given without simultaneously monitored mean arterial blood pressure (MABP) and $PaCO_2$ are worthless. The normal cerebral perfusion discloses the regulatory phenomenon called autoregulation i.e. cerebral circulation will be maintained unchanged despite changes of the perfusion pressure (mainly determined by MABP) within wide limits. This mechanism may easily be disturbed or even completely abolished by pathological processes or pharmacological action. Such impairment of autoregulation may be either global (hemispheric) and/or focal (regional). Using multiple channel equipment and initial slope analysis for repeated CBF measurements in a patient in whom the cerebral perfusion pressure is varied (pharmacologically induced moderate hypertension is most reliable) invariably discloses impairment of autoregulation when present (Fig. 6).

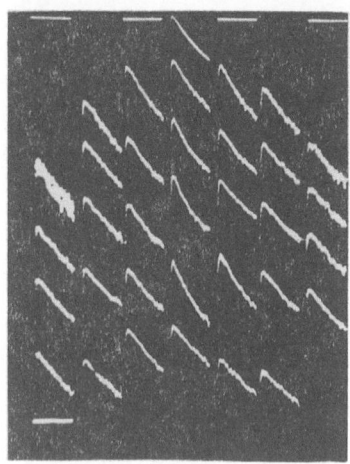 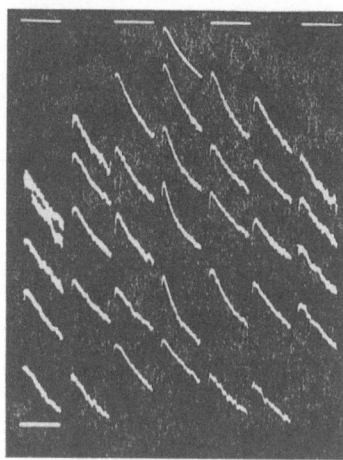

MABP 100 mm Hg
$PaCO_2$ 38 mm Hg
: compare the original photograph.

MABP 120 mm Hg
$PaCO_2$ 39 mm Hg

Fig. 6. Test of cerebral vasomotor function using the apparatus illustrated in Fig. 5. Comparison of the two photographs discloses that increase of MABP ($PaCO_2$ unchanged) is followed by steeper (and more bent) curves in many regions indicating a flow increase i.e. regional loss of autoregulation.

The other main factor influencing the cerebral vasomotion is the CO_2-response: increasing $PaCO_2$ causes vasodilatation and CBF increase and vice versa. In the $PaCO_2$ interval from 20 to 60 mm Hg some have found a linear relationship between $PaCO_2$ and CBF whereas others have found an exponential increase of CBF (13). Using the Kety–Schmidt method a CBF change of 4.5 per cent per mm Hg $PaCO_2$ change has been found. The $CBF_{initial}$ is changed 4 per cent per mm Hg. But there are large differences between the carbon dioxide reactivity in different patients. Thus, correction of two subsequent flow studies, to make them comparable despite $PaCO_2$ differences, is justified only when the $PaCO_2$ change is less than 5 mm Hg and no focal flow abnormalities or increased intracranial pressure are present. To reveal focal abnormalities induced changes of $PaCO_2$ may be useful.

CONCLUSION

The currently available CBF methods have given us a much better understanding of the physiology of the brain and pathophysiological states in man. Anaesthesiologists who are administering potent drugs, many of which are influencing the cerebral perfusion profoundly, have a special interest in CBF studies. All aspects of neuroanaesthesia should be based upon investigations employing a CBF method.

REFERENCES

1. Lennox, W. G. & Gibbs, E. L., The blood flow in the brain and the leg of man, and the changes induced by alteration of blood gases. *J. clin. Invest.* 11, 1155 (1932).
2. Kety, S. S. & Schmidt, C. F., The determination of cerebral blood flow in man by the use of nitrous oxide in low concentrations. *Amer. J. Physiol.* 143, 53 (1945).
3. Kety, S. S. & Schmidt, C. F., The nitrous oxide method for the quantitative determination of cerebral blood flow in man: theory, procedure, and normal values. *J. clin. Invest.* 27, 476 (1948).
4. Zierler, K. L., Theory of the use of arteriovenous concentration differences for measuring metabolism in steady and non-steady states. *J. clin. Invest.* 40, 2111 (1961).
5. Lassen, N. A. & Munck, O., The cerebral blood flow in man determined by the use of radioactive krypton. *Acta physiol. scand.* 33, 30 (1955).
6. Lassen, N. A. & Ingvar, D. H., The blood flow of the cerebral cortex determined by radioactive krypton 85. *Experientia (Basel)* 17, 42 (1961).
7. Ingvar, D. H. & Lassen, N. A., Regional blood flow of the cerebral cortex determined by krypton 85. *Acta physiol. scand.* 54, 325 (1962).
8. Lassen, N. A., Høedt–Rasmussen, K., Sørensen, S. C., Skinhøj, E., Cronquist, S., Bodforss, B. & Ingvar, D. H., Regional cerebral blood flow in man determined by krypton 85. *Neurology (Minneap.)* 13, 719 (1963).

9. Zierler, K. L., Equations for measuring blood flow by external monitoring of radio-isotopes. *Circulat. Res.* 16, 309 (1965).
10. Lassen, N. A. & Høedt–Rasmussen, K., Human cerebral blood flow measured by two inert gas techniques: comparison of the Kety–Schmidt method and the intra-arterial injection method. *Circulat. Res.* 19, 681 (1966).
11. Høedt–Rasmussen, K., Sveinsdottir, E. & Lassen, N. A., Regional cerebral blood flow in man determined by intra-arterial injection of radioactive inert gas. *Circulat. Res.* 18, 237 (1966).
12. Paulson, O. B., Cronquist, S., Risberg, J. & Jeppesen, F. I., Regional cerebral blood flow: a comparison of 8-detector and 16-detector instrumentation. *J. nucl. Med.* 10, 164 (1969).
13. Olesen, J., Paulson, O. B. & Lassen, N. A., Regional cerebral blood flow in man determined by the initial slope of the clearance of intra-arterially injected 133 Xe. *Stroke* 2, 519 (1971).
14. Sveinsdottir, E. & Lassen, N. A., A 256 detector system for measuring regional cerebral blood flow (abstract). *Stroke* 4, 365 (1973).

COMPUTERS

COMPUTER MODELS OF HALOTHANE ANESTHESIA: APPLICATION LEADING TO SERVO-ANESTHESIA

J. E. W. BENEKEN, M. E. SLUIJTER AND J. A. BLOM

INTRODUCTION

In 1950 Bickford (1) described a system for automatic encephalografic control of general anesthesia. The system was used in conjunction with an intravenous injection of pentothal sodium. More recently Franklin and Utter (2) described a parameter identification scheme for EEG data taken during anesthesia. Their analysis is based on a combined autoregressive and moving average description of the EEG wave form. They expect to construct a useful alarm system based on the state of the central nervous system. A reflexcontrolled automatic anesthesia device is described by Hakansson and Malcus (3) in which they used the rectified EMG signal which operates a syringe filled with nembutal and which is connected to an intra-venous catheter. Nerve stimulus occurred once every ten seconds and both the integrated EMG signal and the beak twitch of seagulls was recorded; this technique is reported as being in use for over one year.

Mitamura, Mikami, Sugawara and Yoshimoto (4) and Mitamura, Mikami and Yamamoto (5) have reported on automatic control of respirators. They use mixed expiratory carbon dioxide tension and an ear lobe oximeter to estimate the arterial oxygen tension. Experiments were performed using dogs which were subjected to venous CO_2 loading. The authors claim that this system can only operate under deep anesthesia, since spontaneous breathing is not allowed. A complete systems analysis was performed by Smith and Schwede (6). They applied sinusoidally varying inspired halothane concentrations and recorded the resulting arterial pressure variations. Based on phase-plane studies they constructed a control system for halothane anesthesia in which the arterial pressure was used as the controlled variable. Although the system operated satisfactorily, the authors recognized that optimal control requires more than one variable. Coles, Brown and Lampard (7) describe a system for simultaneous control of respiration and anesthesia. Carbon dioxide, oxygen and tidal volume are used to control the respirator; deviations from a preset blood pressure are used for the control of the anesthetic. Experiments were performed on healthy sheep. No reference was made to pathologic circulatory or respiratory functions. Bartlett (8) described the development of an automated anesthesia machine which will operate in three different modes.

1. The patient breathing on his own (unassisted)
2. The patient determines the respiratory rate, the respirator determines the depth of ventilation (assisted)
3. The respirator controls the ventilation of the patient entirely including occasional deep breaths (controlled)

No results were reported.

A theoretical approach describing the use of a 'Turing' machine for anesthesia control is presented by Stahl (9). An interesting aspect of this study is that the control system operates without a memory. A practical follow up of this approach has not been found.

The references mentioned so far all refer to actual or potential closed loop operation. Off-line prediction of optimal doses for combined infusion-inhalation of ether was described by Seagrave, Zwart, Beneken and Crul (10). A nomogram was constructed based on computer model studies. A clinical test has still to be performed.

Most of the above described on-line systems are based on phenomenological relations and experimental results; they follow a heuristic approach. It is possible, however, that much more can be gained from additional physiological insight. Metabolic acidosis abolishes the response of the myocardium to endogeneously secreted catecholamines. As a result of this, the patient is deprived of his natural compensatory mechanism, e.g. in response to a reduction in circulating blood volume. The awareness of acidosis as a possible cause of a hypotension eliminates the need for continuously monitoring blood gas values and an intravenous administration of sodium bicarbonate may restore the patients cardiac output rapidly. This example was used by DeLand and Maloney (11) to stress the point that improved monitoring equipment needs to be combined with studying patients under operation and application of general physiological principles.

The present paper describes a simple uptake and distribution model for halothane in normal humans. This model is used to illustrate the limitations of servo-anesthesia using simple straightforward control methods. The same model will be used to describe a new method based on the description of the patients state (Blom (12, 13)) and which by-passes some of the earlier disadvantages. Possible implementation that may lead to servo-anesthesia will be indicated.

MULTICOMPARTMENT-MODEL

The model is depicted in Fig. 1. Besides a compartment representing the anesthesia machine and respirator, separate compartments are used to represent the lungs, arterial and mixed venous blood and nine tissue beds in the systemic circulation. This model is adopted from Zwart, Smith and Beneken (14) and the same numerical data were used. For the moment we will limit the discussion to the effect of one anesthetic: halothane.

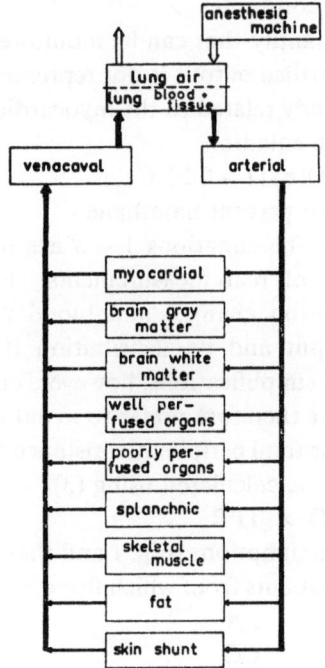

Fig. 1. Block diagram of uptake and distribution model. Each compartment represents a resistor-condensor combination the product of which equals

$$\tau = \frac{\lambda_b V_b + \lambda_t V_t}{\lambda_b q_b}$$ where λ_b and λ_t are partition coefficients of blood and tissues, respectively, and V_b and V_t the respective volumes of blood in the compartment and in the tissue that is assumed to be in equilibrium with blood. This blood flows with a rate q_b through this compartment.

Servo-anesthesia is based on measuring a number of variables that represent the functioning of important physiologic sub-systems. Except for expired concentrations, anesthetic concentrations in other compartments are very difficult to monitor on a routine base. However, information is becoming available about the relation between EEG and halothane concentrations (15). Hakansson et al (3) indicated the power of the EMG in servo-anesthesia. Thus, we assume that brain gray matter concentration C_{bg} is represented by a signal EE derived from the electroencephalogram according to

$$EE = a + bC_{bg} \tag{1}$$

and that a suitable electromyogram signal EM can be derived that is related to the skeletal muscle concentration C_m according to

$$EM = c + dC_m \tag{2}$$

where a, b, c, and d are constants.

Cardiac output is a quantity that can be monitored continuously (Wesseling et al. (16)). Since cardiac output is not represented in the model shown in figure 1, it is in this study related to the myocardial concentration C_{my} (in percent) by the following equation

$$CO = CO(o) (1 - 0.25 \, C_{my}) \tag{3}$$

CO(o) is the value at zero percent halothane.

It will be evident that the equations 1 – 3 are much more complicated when describing results of real measurements. Furthermore interaction between local concentration changes and blood flow is present and the changes in cardiac output and its distribution influence the size of all compartments (14). The simplifications, however, do not invalidate the conclusions to be reached; we therefore prefer to avoid unnecessary complexity. When TPR represents the total peripheral resistance to blood flow, the mean arterial pressure PA can be calculated using (3):

$$PA = CO \times TPR \tag{4}$$

Within the limits of the assumptions, Fig. 1 and the extension with equations 1 through 4 represent a patients from which five quantities can be monitored:
— arterial pressure   PA
— cardiac output   CO
— expired concentration   EC
— electroencephalogram   EE
— electromyogram   EM

Figure 2 shows the responses of these 5 variables to a sudden step in inspired halothane concentration from 0 – 2%.

STRAIGHT FORWARD CONTROL AND ITS LIMITATIONS

In this simple model the only quantity that can be varied to perform a control action is the inspired concentration. When arterial pressure is used as controlled quantity, figure 3 depicts the system. A deviation from the set point causes a change in oxygen flow through the vaporizer (e.g. copper kettle). With some delay, represented by a single compartment, the change in inspired concentration enters the model.

The response of the system from figure 3 to a step-change in the set point value of the arterial pressure from 100 to 50 mm Hg is shown in figure 4.

The required value of the mean arterial pressure is reached after approximately 10 minutes and is properly maintained afterwards. To obtain this response, the inspired concentration (lower tracing) is controlled in a rather oscillatory fashion. By reducing the gain to 0.5 its previous value, the oscillatory behaviour can be reduced, however, at the expense of an increased final error (from 5 to 10 %). Further reduction of the gain down to 0.1 of the original value caused a final error of 30 % of the set point value of the mean arterial pressure: this is undesirable.

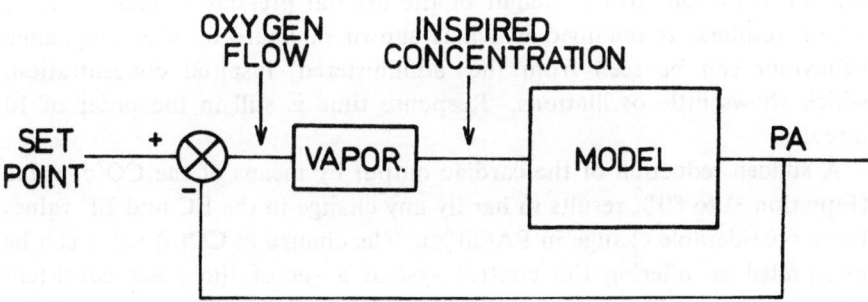

Fig. 3. Block diagram illustrating 'straightforward' control using arterial pressure as the control quantity. The vaporizer and tubing are represented by a single compartment with a time constant of 6 sec.

To investigate the behaviour of this simple control system when the patient's properties would change we again used our model, with the loop gain set at approximately 10 (normal value of Fig. 4). With the anesthesia well underway and stabilized, we increased the total peripheral resistance TPR gradually but irregularly to twice its normal value. It can be seen from figure 5 that the controlled variable, mean arterial pressure, remains almost constant. The inspired concentration reflects the irregularity of the TPR change. Expired and brain gray matter concentrations increased considerably, which may be undesirable in real situations.

A solution could be to incorporate more patient variables in the control system. In the system we are considering only one quantity is available for control, i.e. the inspired concentration. One way to let more patients variables have influence on one single control quantity is to perform a kind of summation, to calculate a weighted average.

As an example, we tried to incorporate the error signals of arterial pressure ΔPA, of expired concentration ΔEC, and a measure for the deviation of the brain gray matter concentration from the required value ΔEE. The weighted average of these three error signals is calculated according to

$$WA = w_1 \Delta PA + w_2 \Delta EC + w_3 \Delta EE \qquad (5)$$

where w_1, w_2 and w_3 are the weighting factors.

It will be obvious that this control system requires the definition of three reference values, one for each of PA, EC and EE. In this model study, the interrelation of these reference values is perfectly known; in patients this will, in general, not be the case.

When consistent reference values are presented, and the relative weight of the concentrations to the weight of the arterial pressure is taken 4 to 1, a step response is obtained which is shown in figure 6. Good dynamic behaviour can be seen from the 'administered' inspired concentration, which shows little oscillations. Response time is still in the order of 10 minutes.

A sudden reduction of the cardiac output by means of the CO(o) value (Equation 3) to 80% results in hardly any change in the EC and EE values but a considerable change in PA(30%). The change in CO(o) value can be interpreted as offering the control system a set of three *not* consistent reference values. The quantity with the smallest weighting factor is sacrificed, which is in this case the arterial pressure PA. Return to normal CO(o) value is rapidly followed by restoration of the previous control levels.

When different weighting values are chosen the response to changes in cardiac output is different. Figure 7 shows this when the relative weight of arterial pressure and concentrations is reversed. Dynamic behaviour is still satisfactory, and now the arterial pressure varies less than in figure 6 (4%) and the concentrations EC and EE show larger variations. The dynamic behaviour appears to be little sensitive to these weight changes.

The limitations of this straight forward control system for servo-anesthesia are now apparent. To attain satisfactory control, one must define the set points for the variables that are incorporated in the control (define the optimal state) and indicate the relative importance of these variables. The overall gain, however, determines the final error that will be present in these variables. The results of the model experiments shown so far illustrate the fact that internal changes in the patient, which interfere with the uptake and distribution properties of the patient, may cause considerable errors. If sufficient information about these internal variations were available continuously, the anesthetist would be kept busy with readjusting gain and weight factors.

This information is not available and furthermore this is no improvement over the present situation where the uninterrupted attention of the anesthetist is required.

SERVO-ANESTHESIA

If there was a way to continuously keep track of the internal changes that take place in a patient and of the effect that these changes have on the relations between the quantities measured from the patient, it should be possible to design a system that controls the level of anesthesia in a perfect way.

If this tracking system (most likely a digital computer) was available, it would certainly need time to become 'acquainted' with the patient. This can be done by looking at the measured quantities and their interrelations when simultaneous changes occur. Sometimes these changes can be provoked by administering certain drugs. Following this learning period the computer will be able to make 'educated guesses' about optimal doses of anesthetic.

The following practical situation can be imagined:

1. the anesthetist starts observation and induction of the patient;
2. all equipment is connected to both patient and computer; the computer starts interpreting the measurements; learning period starts;
3. the anesthetist defines the optimal state of the patient under anesthesia in terms of a series of set points;
4. the computer starts to give suggestions for doses of anesthetic drugs; when these are executed the computer is so informed. When the anesthetist administers a different dose or drug, the computer is also informed. After this 'learning period' the computer gives correct suggestions, which the anesthetist accepts;
5. change to automatic control;
6. in case of emergencies: the computer gives a warning signal; change to

human control; search for cause of alarm and correction of defaults;
7. in case of inconsistencies: the computer tries to diagnose the error, e.g.
   bad electrode contacts; clots in catheter.

If we were sure that in this practical case the whole computer system gave
an immediate warning when it failed and otherwise would act like an
anesthetist, we could say that we reached our goal: servo-anesthesia.

During recent years, control engineers have developed the principle of
'adaptive control' which may prove to be a useful basis for servo-anesthesia.

PRINCIPLES OF ADAPTIVE CONTROL

The dose of anesthetics applied to a patient should depend upon his individual response to these anesthetics. This self evident truth together with the
knowledge that responses not only vary from person to person, but also in
one person from one moment to the other, explains why the anesthetist (or
any control mechanism) should keep track of the patient's response not
only initially but all the time.

Figure 8 shows an adaptive control system. At first, the blocks 'model'
and 'control' contain the *a priori* knowledge we have about our patient,
based on general physiological and anatomical data, body weight and
length and other factors. Both blocks will be updated as soon as information
about this particular patient becomes available by monitoring. Then the
model starts to behave more and more like this patient (it receives the same

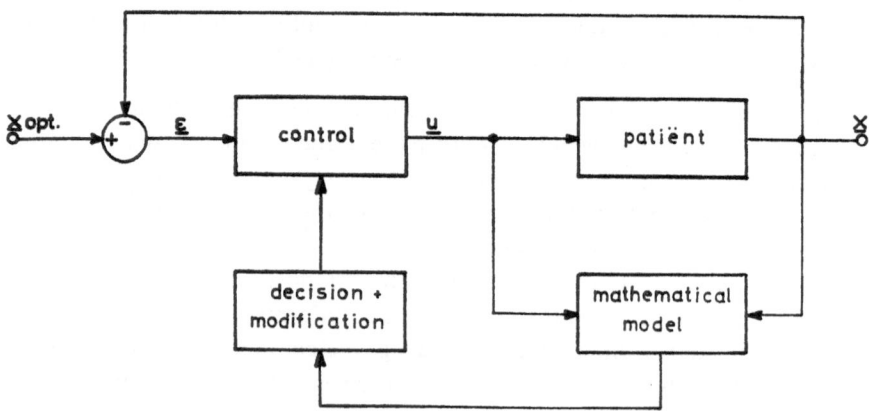

Fig. 8. Adaptive control scheme.
x is patient's state, set of variables measured from patient.
u is control input, set of quantities used to control the patient.
ε difference between required optimal state x_{opt} and actual state x.

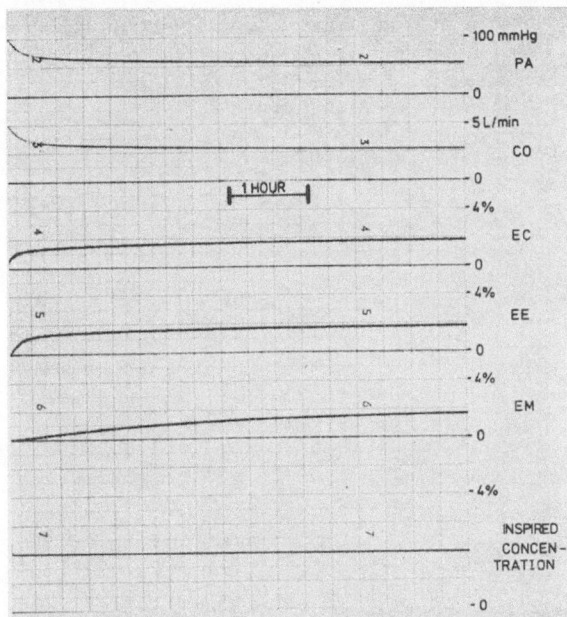

Fig. 2. Response of arterial pressure (PA), cardiac output (CO), expired concentration (EC), 'Electroencephalogram' (EE) and 'Electromyogram' (EM) to sudden increase in inspired halothane concentration from 0-2%. Since constants a and c in equations 1 and 2 are taken equal to zero, and b and d taken equal to unity, scales along the lower 3 channels can be expressed in percent.

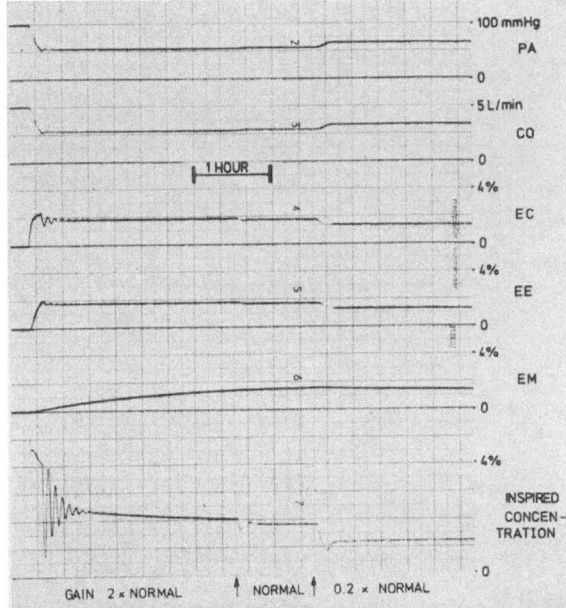

Fig. 4. Patient model controlled in a straightforward manner using arterial pressure as control variable. Step response at twice normal gain; observe increase in final error when gain is reduced. Set point of PA is 50 mm Hg. Maximum inspired halothane concentration is limited.

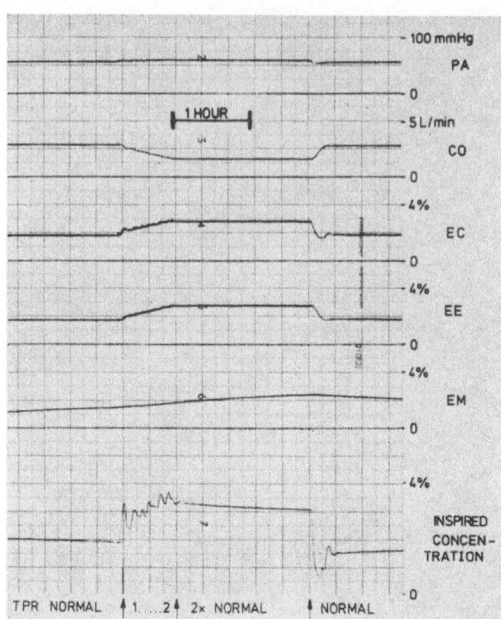

Fig. 5. Similar situation as in fig. 4 with PA as control variable. Between 1 . . . 2, peripheral resistance value TPR is increased from normal to twice normal. Observe error increase in PA and increase in EC and EE levels. Sudden reduction to normal TPR produces no overshoot in PA.

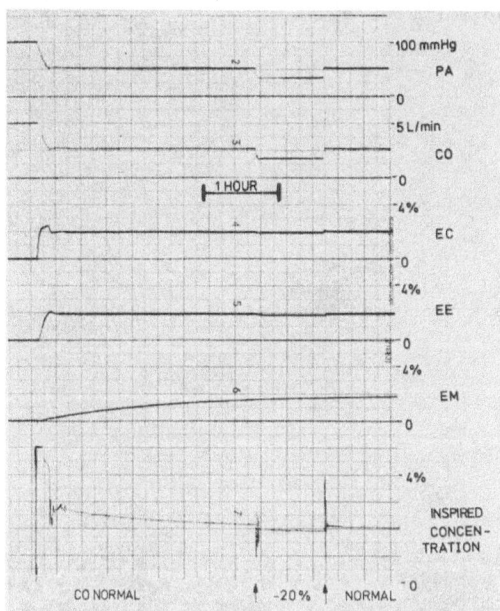

Fig. 6. Step response of patient model to sudden set point change in PA, EC and EE to values corresponding to 2% inspired halothane. Observe little overshoot in PA and EE. Sudden decrease in CO(o) value with 20% causes little variation in EC and EE. PA reduces considerably. Straightforward control with relative values of weight factors $\frac{1}{4}$, 1, 1 for PA, EC and EE respectively.

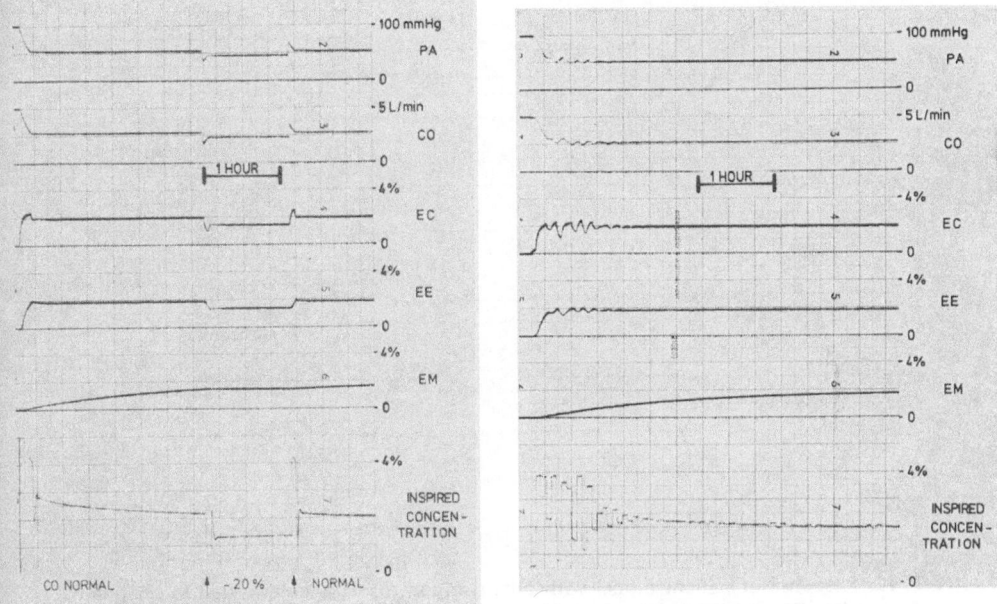

Fig. 7. Similar to fig. 6 except for the relative values of the weight factors: 1, $\frac{1}{4}$, $\frac{1}{4}$ for PA, EC and EE, respectively.
Note little variation of PA in response to CO(o) changes as result of increased 'weight' compared to fig. 6. EC and EE vary much more for the same reason.

Fig. 10. Response to sudden change of PA reference to 50 mm Hg of the patient model controlled by the adaptive control system using PA as control variable. Observe final error that is practically zero.

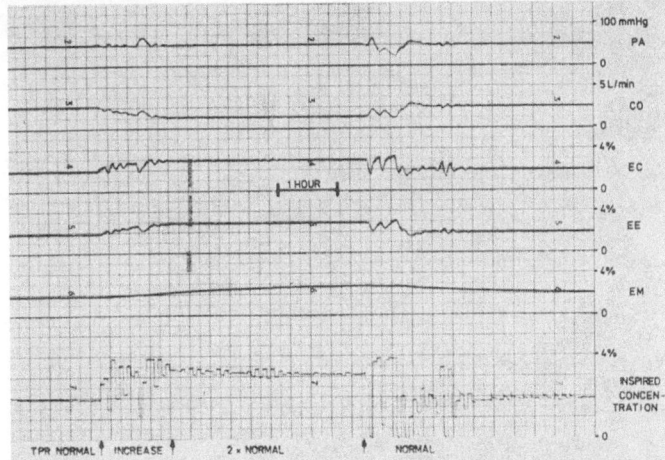

Fig. 11. Similar situation as in fig. 10; adaptive control using PA. Slow increase in peripheral resistance from normal to twice normal, and fast return to normal causes transient irregularities. Final error in PA smaller than 1 %. Inspired concentration levels similar to those in fig. 5.

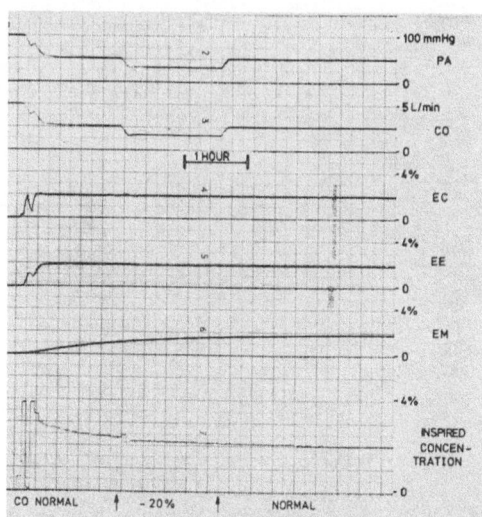

Fig. 12. Response of patient model with adaptive control to a sudden step in set point values of PA, EC and EE; relative weight factors are $\frac{1}{4}$, 1, and 1. Sudden change in CO(o) value has considerable effect on PA value because of low weight factor value. Compare fig. 6.

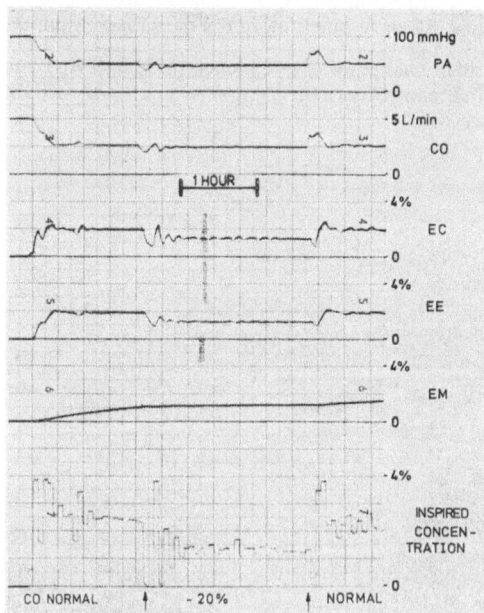

Fig. 13. Similar responses as in fig. 12; weight factors are 1, $\frac{1}{4}$ and $\frac{1}{4}$ for PA, EC and EE respectively. PA error becomes negligible.

inputs), and the control will become optimal for this patient.

In other words: adaptive control is optimal control based on a model, the properties of which are by the best possible means, determined from the patient. (For further details see appendix.)

MATHEMATICAL MODEL

Why do we monitor a patient? Mainly because we want to keep track of all important physiological quantities which might indicate the patient's condition. We may assume for good reasons that all important variables are monitored, and that non-important variables are not. Then we have obtained exactly the set of variables which will be needed as an input to the model. We will call this set of variables: the patient's state. The patient's state may include arterial and venous pressure, heart rate, rate of respiration, electroencephalogram etc.

Now we assume, that we can define an optimal state for this patient, i.e. propose a set of values such that if all monitored variables had these values, the patient would be in the optimal condition (state). Then the purpose of the control is to minimize the difference between optimal and actual variable values. As indicated before, this is only possible if we have a reasonably correct model of the patient. This mathematical model can be obtained by observing both the state variables and the controls and estimating their relationships; these relations are usually called: a mathematical model.

WEIGHT FACTORS

Of course, the criterion for finding the right doses can be changed in such a way that only one variable is forced to the optimal value. This policy may, however, prove to be hazardous. Suppose we use halothane, and try to keep the expired concentration constant. If now in a certain patient the arterial pressure drops much more than had been expected, this might be fatal if not discovered soon enough. Therefore, we would like the arterial pressure to modify the control; i.e. when the arterial pressure moves away from the optimal value, the inspired concentration is decreased automatically. It seems to us illogical, that a variable that is worth monitoring, has no influence over the control of dosage. However, a possibility must be included to rate all monitored variables to their importance in the control. Therefore, weight factors should indicate, how important we think it is to keep a certain variable close to the optimal value.

The decision on what is the optimal state for a particular patient will be based on the anesthetist's experience.

IMPLEMENTATION ON A DIGITAL COMPUTER

The mathematical model, and the control logarithms are very well suited for implementation on a small digital computer. Possibly, few changes would be necessary in the existing monitoring and control equipment. The processing time is so small, that many measurements can be checked and processed every minute, so that even when the computer is in control, emergencies can be detected and reported almost immediately.

The theory of learning systems has progressed so far that, in routine cases, a computer could fulfil most of the tasks the anesthetist has today. On the other hand, we have a sharp awareness of the limitations of adaptive systems, so that we know that in many non-routine cases the computer will never be full-proof.

Yet we believe that the anesthetist will be able to use the computer for the benefit of both himself and the patient.

ADAPTIVE CONTROL, ITS POWER AND LIMITATIONS

The same patient model that was used to show the effect of straightforward control, was controlled adaptively with a Digital Equipment PDP-9 computer, according to figure 9.

This adaptive controller was a rather crude version of the anticipated system, lacking both any security measures and the possibility of human intervention. Moreover adaptation started without any a priori information.

Samples were taken regularly each 4 seconds.* In reality this would be 4 minutes, but could be considerably less if necessary. This is the only disadvantage of a digital controller: where the analog controller is aware of

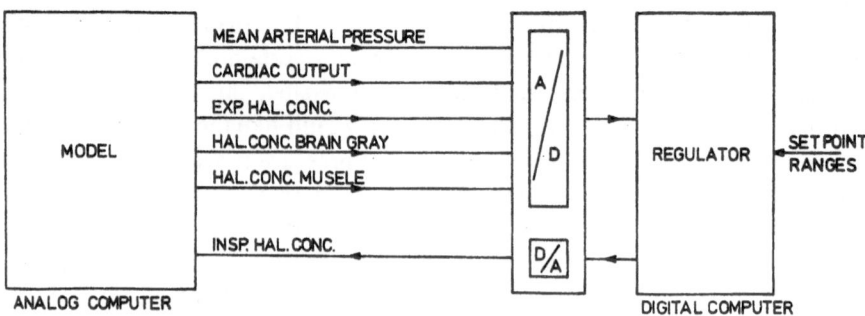

Fig. 9. Adaptive control of a patient model.

* To reduce experimentation time, the patient model operated at a 60 times increased time scale.

all state variable values at all times and can change its output instantaneously, the digital computer's output is constant during the sample interval.

As the essential features of adaptive control we expect:

1. a period of learning, both immediately following the start and after a sudden change in the patient's parameters; in both cases co-operation with the anesthetist can be necessary, which possibility is excluded in this model study;
2. satisfactory control once a reasonable model of the patient's system is obtained.

The response of the adaptive control system to a step change in set point value of the arterial pressure from 100 to 50 mm Hg is shown in figure 10. Since no *a priori* information is available to the controller, first a 'trial input' is given (20% of maximum). After 4 minutes the results are available and a maximum halothane percentage (4%) is inspired. After 4 more minutes again the maximum is inspired, after which the set point value is reached in a slightly oscillatory way. After 12 minutes 60 mm Hg is reached, after which the final error decreases to *less than 1%*. Had the 'trial input' been the maximum (4%), possibly if *a priori* information was available, then control would have been almost 4 min. faster. Note the similarity of this figure to figure 4.

To test the adaptation of the controller the total peripheral resistance TPR was gradual increased to twice its normal value. Figure 11 shows that after some oscillations the final error in AP is less than 1%. All other variables behave in the same way as in figure 5. After some time TPR is suddenly returned to its normal value. Here the weakness of adaptive controllers shows: if the patient's system has a fast and drastic change in its parameters, it takes some time to 'unlearn' and adapt again. At one time the arterial pressure reaches a low 25 mm Hg, which is highly undesirable. Had more *a priori* information been built in, this would not have happened. But again the final error is less than 1%.

For reasons indicated earlier, in addition to the arterial pressure, both the expired halothane concentration and the brain compartment were allowed to influence the controller. Figure 12 gives the response of the controller, if EC and EE are weighted four times more than PA. Unlike figure 6 the final error is almost zero. When CO was suddenly reduced 20% the control hardly changed because EC and EE did not change. Therefore the decreased value of PA was not counteracted. When CO resumed its normal value the control hardly changed either.

Figure 13 shows the same, but now PA is considered four times as important as EC and EE. Now, after a 20% decrease of CO, PA resumed almost
its normal value while EC and EE are lowered.

Again it must be emphasized that this realization of an adaptive controller
is far from perfect. First of all, the sampling interval was too long in this
simulation, due to the time scale change of the patient model, but in actual
clinical work it could be shortened appreciably. Second, and more fundamental is the bad behaviour of adaptive systems if large changes in values
occur rapidly. This situation is handled best by a straightforward type of
controller, or an adaptive controller with a simpler structure. Future
research, therefore, will include a study of parallel operations of different
types of controller in such a way that the advantages of the adaptive controller are retained while its weakness may be diminished to a considerable
extent.

DISCUSSION

The results and conclusions arrived at so far are based on attempts to control
a multi-compartment model of human uptake and distribution properties
for halothane. This model is very much simplified and neglects many important aspects that play a role during anesthesia. The effects of carbon
dioxide on cardiac output and its interference with the halothane effect on
the brain is not represented. The magnitude of these influences may be
relatively small. However, in studies concerning gain of control systems,
slight changes may have large effects.

Also, the magnitude of the responses on halothane concentration variations may be in error. It was a rather arbitrary assumption, based on
overall figures (14) that with 2% inspired halothane the arterial pressure
would be reduced to one-half normal at equilibrium.

The authors are well aware of these and other limitations of this patient
model. However, it was used as a first step to evaluate the possibilities for
servo-anesthesia and to distinguish between two types of control techniques:
straightforward control and adaptive control. The simple model used so far
served this purpose so that a more complicated model was unnecessary in
this first stage.

Controlling anesthesia with only one variable (inspired concentration) is
also not very realistic, but was useful at this stage.

The next step will be to extend the computer model to allow for control
of both respiration and anesthetic administration. Comparing control
techniques on such a model will sharpen up the distinction between the two.

What are the objectives that one has in mind in designing a servo-anesthesia system?

Although not a complete listing, the following points are important:

- reaching the required anesthetic level in the brain after minimal time
- the absence of severe overshoots; in other words, critical damping of oscillations
- being able to handle more than one control variable
- controlling properties should be insensitive for internal changes in the patient that interact with the uptake and distribution properties
- controlling properties should be little or not dependent on inter-individual differences; i.e., little *a priori* knowledge needed.
- anesthetist should only be called in when real and unexpected emergencies occur.

The feasibility study performed so far does not touch on all these points.

Straightforward control is simple, easy to implement and has good dynamic properties. The static properties are less ideal in that considerable final errors remain when the loop gain is too low. This is a result of the fact that the final error is proportional to the percentage of inspired concentration.

The final error could be reduced considerably if an integrating controller was used. In these cases the inspired concentration would be adjusted proportional to the integral of the final error. This has been tried using the present patient model but resulted in severe instabilities (oscillations) caused by the additional phase lag that was introduced in the control loop. The major limitation of the straightforward control approach is that internal changes of the patient remain unrecognized, and therefore cannot be corrected. This leads to unexpected large final errors, unless the anesthetist adjusts the gain controls continuously. This is what servo-anesthesia tries to avoid.

The adaptive control approach is less simple, requires a (small) digital computer, and in this study the dynamic properties are slightly less than with proprtional control. The major advantage of adaptive control is that it produces final errors that are essentially equal to zero. Slow changes in the patient's state are followed and the error kept at zero.

It is expected that in more complicated model studies and in animal studies the adaptive control system will behave much more reliably than the straightforward control, especially when more than one quantity is to be controlled. The learning process can be hastened considerably when, for example, the parameter of the previous, or an 'average' patient are used as initial estimates in the mathematical model of the adaptive control system. After applying this control system to a large number of patients, it may prove possible to calculate multiple regression relations between the parameters of the parameter matrices A and B (appendix) and simple data such as weight, length, age, sex, and occupational habits.

Once reliable estimates of the parameter values for a particular patient are obtained it is extremely likely that several of them have physiological or anatomical correlates which otherwise could not be determined. This may support or extend diagnosis using other means. Particularly interesting is this application with respect to trend detection. Slow variations in the patient's state may be detected using this technique; this leads itself to application to patients in the intensive care unit where procedures are not much different:

– a need to define the optimal state – a number of therapeutic means (e.g. drugs) to reach this state-monitoring by the computer of the relevant state variables.

Some of these considerations, on the applications of adaptive control are speculative. However, we feel that the results obtained so far are good enough to continue this study. This continuation will be along the lines presented in this chapter. After more extensive computer model studies, the system will be tested during animal studies. When promising results have been obtained, clinical studies will be performed. There, the anesthetist will remain in the control loop; the computer will make suggestions and the anesthetist will decide whether to follow up these suggestions or to ignore them. Once the system has proven to be reliable on a great many patients and under widely varying circumstances, we plan to start developing the necessary hardware such as sensors and controllers. Only then will we be able to specify these requirements. The continuation of this study is a challenge to both anesthesiologists and engineers; close co-operation between them will bear fruitful results.

ACKNOWLEDGEMENT
Ir. D. H. Bekkering is greatly acknowledged for initiating the research to supply a mathematical basis for physiological processes. F. Lioni assisted skilfully in compiling relevant references. A. Zwart and A. van Dieren were indispensable in setting up the computer model.

APPENDIX
Formal definition of state variable:

A state variable is a variable, having a numerical value and giving information about the patient. It may be given an obvious name, and may have an obvious dimension.

Examples of state variables are:

length	value e.g.	185 (cm)
heart rate		98 (beats/min)
systolic pressure		142 (mm Hg)
expired halothane concentration		1.8 (%)

The EEG-signal is more complex. It must be broken down into several state variables, each having a numerical value. One state variable might be the dominant frequency. This breaking up of complex information into units, the state variables, can always be done.

Now we can formalize the patient's *state:*

By the state of a patient is meant the minimum set of state variables, which contains sufficient information about the past history of the patient to uniquely describe his condition and – provided we know the ways the state variables interact and the control forces that we will apply in the future – to compute this state at any time in the future.

This definition has many implications (13), but the two most important implications are:

1. we want to predict the patient's future state.
2. prediction is only possible if we measure the minimum set of state variables and know the ways they interact.

Now construct the patient's state to include all variables that will change, or may change, during anesthesia in some ordered way. Choose one variable and call it x_1, choose a second and call it x_2 and so on. If we have a total of n variables we have:

$$\underline{x} = \begin{bmatrix} x_1 \\ x_2 \\ \cdot \\ \cdot \\ \cdot \\ x_n \end{bmatrix}, \text{ where } \underline{x} \text{ is the state vector.}$$

Now choose a coordinate system. Align x_1 along the x-axis, x_2 along the y-axis and so on. Then the state represents a point in an n-dimensional space. By observing $\underline{x}$ for some time, plotting it in this n-dimensional space, we have a means to follow movements of the patient's state.

Likewise we can define the *optimal state* $\underline{x}_{opt}$:

The optimal state is the state the anesthetist wants the patient to be in.

It can be envisaged as a point or a region in the n-dimensional space. If the patient's state is within this region, his state is optimal and cannot be improved, if it is outside the optimal region, something should be done to move the state into the optimal region.

For this purpose control forces are available: inspiration of halothane, oxygen, carbon dioxide, injection of muscle relaxants, heating etc. By ordering the control forces in some way we construct

$$\underline{u} = \begin{bmatrix} u_1 \\ u_2 \\ \cdot \\ \cdot \\ \cdot \\ u_m \end{bmatrix}, \text{ where } \underline{u} \text{ is the control vector.}$$

When we describe the interactions between the state variables and the control forces, we obtain a dynamic model of the patient. Note that at the moment we only want a general, qualitative description of these relations.

Suppose all variable values are measured at discrete intervals, T seconds apart. Then we can write

$$x_1(t+T) = a_{10} + a_{11}x_1(t) + a_{12}x_2(t) + \ldots\ldots + a_{1n}x_n(t)$$
$$+ b_{11}u_1(t) + b_{12}u_2(t) + \ldots\ldots + b_{1m}u_m(t) + w_1(t),$$

which states that x_1 at time $t+T$ depends on all the previous values of x_1,

$x_2, \ldots \ldots x_n$ and $u_1, u_2 \ldots \ldots u_m$, and that the momentary uncertainty in this relation is w_1. For all other state variables we can derive a similar expression. Combining these we may write in matrix notation

$x(t+T) = a_0 + Ax(t) + Bu(t) + w(t)$,

which formula states that we expect interrelations between every x_i and u_i component, with some uncertainties w_i due to interactions of variables that we did not or could not include in the state vector.

Now suppose a_0, A and B are known, and that we just measured $x(t)$. Then $u(t)$ remains to be chosen such that $x(t+T)$ will be as close to the optimal state as is possible. But $x(t+T)$ is not known yet, due to the uncertainty term $w(t)$. The best prediction for $x(t+T)$ is

$\hat{x}(t+T) = a_0 + Ax(t) + Bu(t)$,

and now it is possible to calculate the optimal control force, such that it minimizes $//x_{opt} - x(t+T)//^2$ (13).

We now drop the supposition that a_0, A and B are known. Then their values need to be determined. Procedures exist to find estimates $\hat{a}_0$, $\hat{A}$ and $\hat{B}$ of a_0, A and B which give a best fit to the observed state variable values (13). This means, that it is only necessary to observe the patient for some time to obtain a unique model, accurately adapted to this individual patient. If the patient is kept under constant observation (as is done already by monitoring) it is possible at all times to have a 'best', constantly updated model, which allows predictions of his state in the future and the calculations of an optimal anesthesia.

REFERENCES

1. Bickford, R. G., Automatic electroencephalographic control of general anesthesia. *EEG Clin. Neurophysiol.* 2, 93-96 (1950).
2. Franklin, G. F. & Utter, D. H., Parameter identification from EEG data taken during anesthesia. *Proc. 5th Hawaii International Conference on System Sciences*, Western Periodicals Co. 15-17 (1972).
3. Hakansson, C. H. & Malcus, B., A reflex-controlled automatic anesthesia device for animal use. *Phys. Med. Biol.* 14, 559-562 (1969).
4. Mitamura, Y., Mikami, T., Sugawara, H. & Yoshimoto, C., An optimally controlled respirator. *IEEE Trans. BME*, 18, 330-332 (1971).
5. Mitamura, Y., Mikami, T. & Yamamoto, K., A dual control system of artificial respiration. *Proc. Xth ICMBE Dresden* (1973).
6. Smith, N. T. & Schwede, H. D., The response of arterial pressure to halothane: A system analysis. *Med. & Biol. Engng* 10, 207-221 (1972).
7. Coles, J. R., Brown, W. A. & Lampard, D. G., Computer control of respiration and anesthesia. *Med. & Biol. Engng* 11, 262-267 (1973).

8. Bartlett, R. B., Automated Anesthesia Machine. *Medical Instrumentation* 7/1 (1973).
9. Stahl, W. R., A programmed automaton for anesthesia control. *Med. Electron & Biol. Engng*, 3, 389-401 (1965).
10. Seagrave, R. C., Zwart, A., Beneken, J. E. W. & Crul, J. F., Optimization of combined infusion-inhalation ether anesthesia. *Proc. Xth ICMBE Dresden*, 24-8 (1973).
11. DeLand, E. C. & Maloney, J. V., Physiologic monitoring in the operating room. *Bull. Amer. Coll. Surgeons* 55 (1970).
12. Blom, J. A., Analyse van fysiologische systemen, *De Ingenieur*, 85, 666-669 (1973).
13. Blom, J. A., Analysis of physiological systems by parameter estimation techniques. *T.H.-report* 73-E-36, *ISBM* 90 6144 036X. Technological University, Eindhoven.
14. Zwart, A., Smith, N. T. & Beneken, J. E. W., Multiple model approach to uptake and distribution of halothane: The use of an analog computer. *Computers & Biomed. Res.*, 5, 228-238 (1972).
15. Lopes da Silva, F. H., Smith, N. T., Zwart, A. & Nichols, W. W., Spectral analysis of the EEG during Halothane anesthesia: input-output relations. *Enceph. & Clin. Neurophysiol.*, 33, 311-319 (1972).
16. Wesseling, K. H., Smith, N. T., Nichols, W. W., Weber, J. A. P., Wit, B. de & Beneken, J. E. W., Beat-to-beat cardiac output from the aortic pressure pulse contour. Boerhaave course 'Measurement in anesthesia', Leiden (1973).

COMPUTERIZED MEASUREMENTS IN ANAESTHESIA

J. A. LACK

The purpose of a computer facility in an operating room is to provide a 'backup' monitoring service to the anaesthetist, a watchdog to keep an eye on physiological variables which may change without overt clinical signs. It also allows the calculation of variables which would not otherwise be practical in a clinical setting. These range from trivial to exotic, but the important advantage that a computer has to offer is the capability of integrating these results into a general picture of the systems being monitored.

The computer must be the 'Gentleman's gentleman' – always ready but never intruding. It must run with a minimum of attention and absolute reliability. Reliability is perhaps the most important quality demanded of all the equipment used for clinical monitoring, not just the computer; we are continually faced with the problem of choosing between reliability and additional refinements (often in the name of accuracy), but there are few physiological measurements that have to be made to a better accuracy than $\pm$ 5 per cent and usually $\pm$ 10 per cent is adequate. By use of a computer, a measurement with an individual accuracy of 10 per cent can be repeated 10 times and the results averaged to give a more reliable mean. This can be achieved without additional trouble to the anaesthetist.

When considering what measurements to make in the operating room, the anaesthetist must first decide what will help most in the care of the patient.

Essentially, he is trying to achieve two things; to prevent harm befalling his patients and to obtain an indication of what therapeutic measures may be necessary at any given time.

To protect patients as far as possible, it is appropriate to examine the commonest factors involved in anaesthetic morbidity. One of the best accounts of this comes from Australia (1), where 286 deaths of patients, where anaesthetic complications may have been responsible, were investigated. The factors involved in each death were then analysed. Monitoring efforts and measurements should be directed towards eliminating these factors as far as possible. For example, secondary variables such as the electrocardiogram have been monitored in the past when it might be more appropriate to concentrate more on those aspects which will cause changes in the electrocardiogram to occur. The measurements chosen to be discussed are ordered according to the priorities dictated by this mortality study (1). The emphasis is placed on basic or simple measurements that should be relatively trouble-free in a realistic working environment, and should not involve the anaesthetist's time once the anaesthetic has been started. Table 1 is derived from Holland's results and lists the ten most common factors contributing to anaesthetic mortality, and the percentage of deaths to which each contributed. It was found that four or five factors were usually present in any given death where anaesthesia might be held responsible. Some of these categories are very broad and some are not preventable by intraoperative monitoring, but nevertheless they should be borne in mind when according priorities to a monitoring system.

Table 1. Factors contributing to anaesthetic deaths.

Factors present in	% of 286 Deaths
Inadequate ventilation	55
Inadequate assessment of fluid balance during operation	55
Inadequate assessment of fluid balance before operation	52
Inadequate management of crisis	49
Overdosage	41
Inadequate observation of patient	33
Technical mishap	23
Incorrect reversal of muscle relaxants	22
Inadequate postoperative supervision	19
Inhalation of vomit	17
Derived from Med. J. Aust. *1* : 12, 573 (1970).	

VENTILATION

There are two fundamental facts that must be known when assessing ventilation; the amount of oxygen going to the patient, and the amount of carbon dioxide being cleared from the patient.

Obviously many other factors are concerned in the quality of ventilation, but these two are of prime interest. For these measurements one needs a pneumotachograph and a rapid responding carbon dioxide analyser. It is also desirable for the airway pressure to be monitored in patients being ventilated, and for this one requires a pressure transducer: this latter will allow the measurement of compliance. The most practical measurement of this variable for routine operating room use is static end-inspiratory compliance. This is obtained by dividing the volume at end-inspiration by the pressure at that time.

The expired volume of carbon dioxide is the instantaneous product of the expired concentration of carbon dioxide and the integral of the output of the pneumotachograph at that time.

$$V_{CO_2} = F_{ECO_2} \cdot V_E \tag{1}$$

The alveolar dead space to tidal volume ratio is derived with the conventional equation.

$$\frac{V_{DALV}}{V_E} = \frac{Pa_{CO_2} - P_{ETCO_2}}{Pa_{CO_2}} \tag{2}$$

The alveolar ventilation may be calculated from

$$\dot{V}_{ALV} = \dot{V}_E \ \frac{P_{\overline{E}CO_2}}{Pa_{CO_2}} \tag{3}$$

If one assumes an RQ of 0.8, then

$$V_{O_2} = 1.25 \ V_{CO_2} \tag{4}$$

and one may approximate that

$$P_{AO_2} = P_{IO_2} - 1.25 \ Pa_{CO_2} \tag{5}$$

End pulmonary capillary oxygen pressure, equal to P_{AO_2}, may be used to calculate end pulmonary capillary oxygen content from the oxy-haemoglobin dissociation curve. From the same curve the arterial and mixed venous oxygen contents are also determined. The degree of shunting may then be calculated using the shunt equation.

$$\frac{Q_s}{Q_t} = \frac{Cc'o_2 - Cao_2}{Cc'o_2 - C\bar{v}o_2} \tag{6}$$

The cardiac output may be derived from the classical Fick equation.

$$Qt = 100 . \frac{V_{O_2}}{Ca_{O_2} - C\bar{v}_{O_2}} \tag{7}$$

The list of what can be calculated extends of course as far as the individual concerned cares to make it; cardiac index, stroke volume, $V_{D\ ANAT}$, $V_{D\ PHYS}$ and work of respiration may be useful in particular situations.

In these calculations a number of assumptions have been made. These allow measurements that are accurate enough for clinical purposes and will evaluate trends in physiological variables: the patient is assumed to be in a steady state; this is difficult to achieve, and to minimise any error it is necessary to average all these calculations over some few minutes. The RQ may not be 0.8, but for operating room use the approximations are close enough.

We have therefore the situation where, by use of a computer and fairly simple measurements, we can calculate the various physiological parameters indicated in Table 2, without distracting the anaesthetist from his observation of the patient.

Table 2. Some variables which may be derived from those measured.

Given				
Airflow	Airway Pressure	CO_2	Pa_{CO_2}	$P\bar{v}_{O_2}$
Calculate				Pa_{O_2}
Tidal volume	Compliance	CO_2	V_D	Q_T
Minute volume		Output	V_A	Q_S/Q_T
I-E Ratio			V_D/V_E	
Rate				

Which of these are practical for daily use? One could reasonably have tidal and minute volumes, I-E ratio and compliance calculations available, with a warning device should the compliance fall outside the range of 20 to 100 ml/cm H_2O.

FLUID BALANCE

Here we have a much more difficult problem, which may start long before surgery, out of reach of our measuring system. The problems of electrolyte

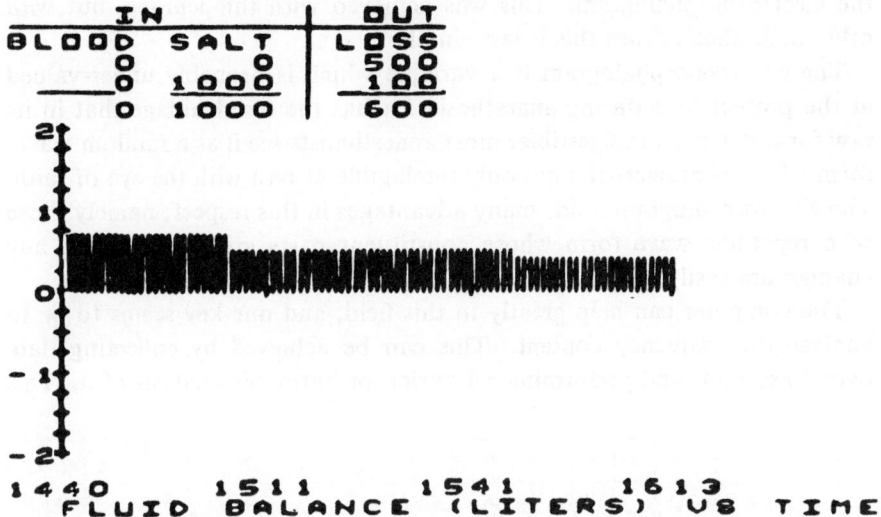

```
     IN            OUT
BLOOD  SALT     LOSS
   0      0      500
   0   1000      100
   0   1000      600
```

Fig. 1. Fluid balance.

imbalance are not soluble on a simple level in the operating room, and we would appear to be limited to a relatively elementary accounting system for fluid balance, together with the central venous pressure when appropriate. Figure 1 is a computer generated chart. One of these may be generated for each category of measurements. For fluid balance there are three main classes – blood transfused, other infusions and blood loss. Occasionally, urine output is included when patients are catheterised. Blood loss is measured by any of the conventional methods and entered manually. Infusions and transfusions are also entered in separate categories and a simple positive-negative balance chart generated.

ELECTROENCEPHALOGRAM
Drugs are often administered intuitively, but there is a very good argument to be made for a more rational approach. The uptake and distribution of anaesthetic agents is a field which has now had much work done in it. For maximum efficiency, the required anaesthetic depth should be reached as rapidly as possible, and then not exceeded. The advantages to the patient are many: toxic side effects of some agents such as methoxyflurane are directly dose related and prolonged recovery times are the inevitable accompaniment of an overdose of anaesthetic. A servo-controlled anaesthetic was given twenty years ago by Bickford (2) utilizing information derived from

the electroencephalogram. This was achieved with thiopentone, but with other anaesthetic drugs this is less simple.

The electroencephalogram is a variable which is probably under-valued at the present time during anaesthesia. It has the disadvantage that in its raw form it is most indigestible; most anaesthetists see it as a random waveform whose characteristics are only intelligible at best with the eye of faith. The electrocardiogram holds many advantages in this respect; namely those of a repetitive wave form whose constituent parts are well defined; any changes are easily recognised.

The computer can help greatly in this field, and one key seems to be to analyse the frequency content. This can be achieved by collecting data over 30 seconds and performing a Fourier, or harmonic analysis of it. This

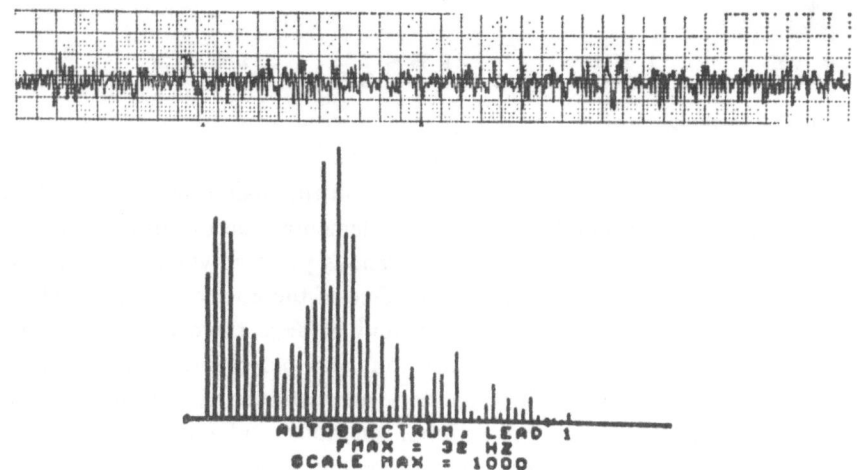

Fig. 2. Frequency content of a strip of electroencephalogram.

will determine the amount of any frequency present in the segment and this can then be displayed as a graph of amplitude against frequency (Figure 2). For the electroencephalogram, frequencies of interest lie up to 24 Hz. These are divided conventionally into four bands; Delta, from 0 - 4 Hz; Theta from 4 - 8 Hz; Alpha from 8 - 12 Hz and Beta from 12 Hz upwards. We have been examining the spectra from patients undergoing halothane anaesthesia with the aims of first, defining the best areas of the brain to record from, and second, defining the changes that may be expected in these areas. In order to do this, we arranged the electrodes on the scalp in the international

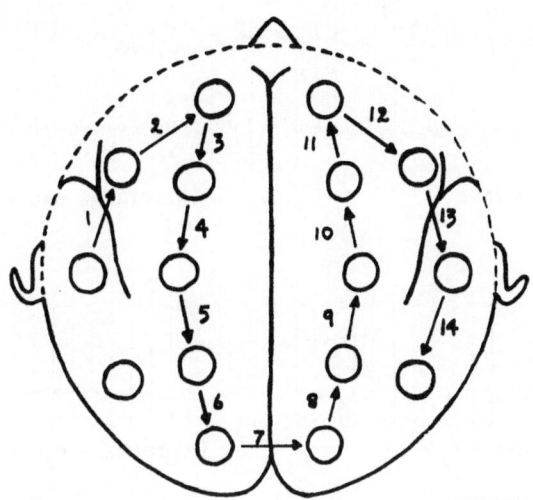

Fig. 3. EEG electrode placement.

10 - 20 system, connected in order such that the voltage difference between any pair of electrodes is the sum of the intervening voltages (Figure 3). We then made a five-minute recording. The patient was given halothane in oxygen to breathe according to the dosage schedule of Lowe (3). After half an hour another recording was made, and blood drawn for gases and an end-expired gas sample analysed for halothane. The inspired gases were then changed to 70% nitrous oxide, 30% oxygen and 1% halothane, and after fifteen minutes another recording made, with CO_2 added to give an arterial partial pressure of 50 mm Hg.

Typical changes in the EEG are shown in figure 4. The raw waveforms do of course hold all the information content, but in a much less evident form. The harmonic analysis of the data shows clear changes (Figure 5). The graphs are of amplitude squared against frequency, 0 - 24 Hz. Each line consists of thirty seconds of data, and every subsequent line is placed behind the first with a slight offset, so that the most recent trace is at the back. The awake trace shows a peak centered around 12 Hz, together with some 2 Hz activity. The halothane trace shows an overall increase in power, together with a slight downward shift in frequency to a peak around 10 Hz. When nitrous oxide is added, there is only one peak, around 1 Hz, and diminishing activity up to 16 Hz. Adding CO_2 to a mean arterial level of 50 mm Hg decreases all frequencies above 2 Hz.

We have now, we hope, a tool which will allow us to read something

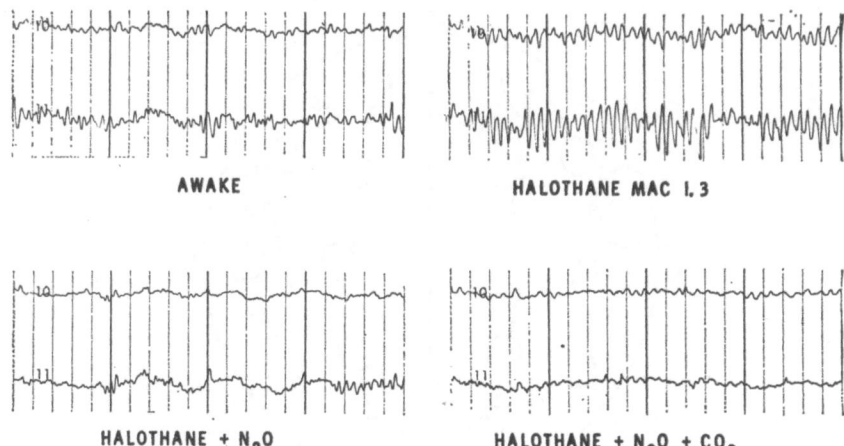

Fig. 4. Raw EEG waveforms.

about cerebral activity presented in an easily assimilated form. The details of the changes that occur with intermediate stages of anaesthesia, and with different anaesthetics, remain to be worked out, as do the best leads to record from. Our preliminary study has defined normal spectra in nine patients, and the changes to be expected under two defined conditions, but this is obviously only the tip of the iceberg. Experience with this clinically in an informal setting has been useful. It has demonstrated on two occasions its ability to show hypoxia before it was clinically apparent, and certainly before the electrocardiogram showed overt changes. It should be possible before long to assess levels of anaesthesia using this technique, and so remove the guesswork frequently responsible for anaesthetic drug overdosage.

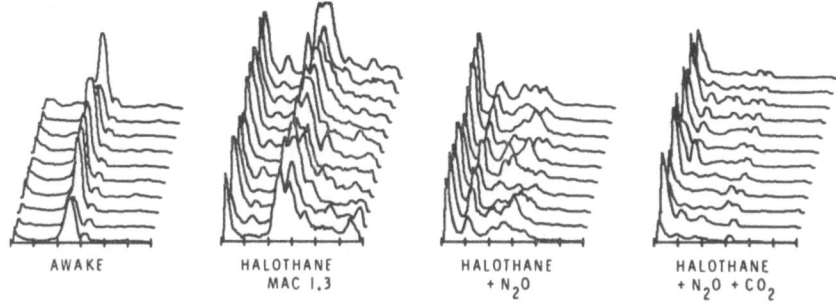

Fig. 5. Spectral analysis of EEG data.

ELECTROCARDIOGRAM

The electrocardiogram is not really very productive of useful, 'therapeutic' information. We have started to look at the ST segment level changes automatically, but there are major programming problems. Waveform classification has been successfully achieved for the QRS complex but not really for the P waves. Figure 6 shows a strip of electrocardiogram. The computer has identified all the QRS complexes and classified them according to shape. The various QRS shapes are shown with an expanded time scale, and their frequencies listed beneath. Probably a non-fade oscilloscope display of the raw waveform is the best value at present.

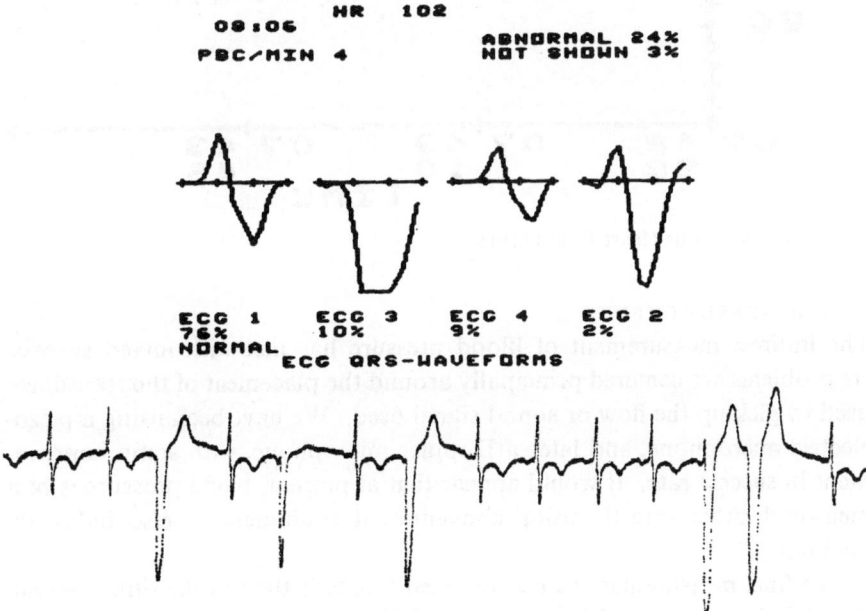

Fig. 6. QRS waveform classification.

INSTANTANEOUS HEART RATE DISPLAY

The advantage of this kind of display over the old-fashioned heart-rate meter is considerable. It shows instantaneously any change in rhythm, and the type of rhythm is often able to be diagnosed rapidly. Figure 7 shows an example of sinus rhythm turning into regular premature beats (upper row) followed by a compensatory pause (lower row), turning to an irregularly irregular pulse (atrial fibrillation).

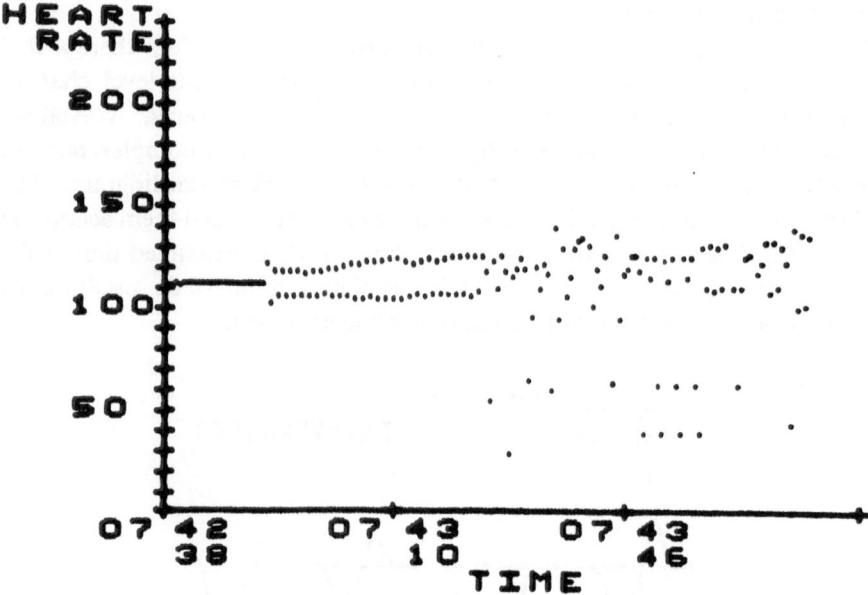

Fig. 7. Instantaneous Heart Rate Display.

OTHER MEASUREMENTS

The indirect measurement of blood pressure has met with mixed success. Its problems are centered principally around the placement of the transducer used to pick up the flow or sound signal used. We have been using a piezo-electric microphone, and later a Doppler microphone, with some improvement in success rate. It would appear that at present, blood pressure is best measured either directly using conventional equipment or else indirectly manually.

The final measurement to be discussed briefly is the systolic time interval. This has been measured in a number of different ways. The simplest is the R-B interval, from the R-wave of the electrocardiogram, to the onset of the brachial pulse wave (Figure 8).

Changes in this interval reflect changes in the contraction time of the left ventricle, though when and why these changes occur is still under much discussion. Figure 9 shows the R-B interval of a 27 year old woman having a laparoscopy. The reason for the sudden increase of R-B interval following nitrous oxide administration is unclear, though negative inotropic cardiac changes due to this drug are described. Subsequently, however, the interval

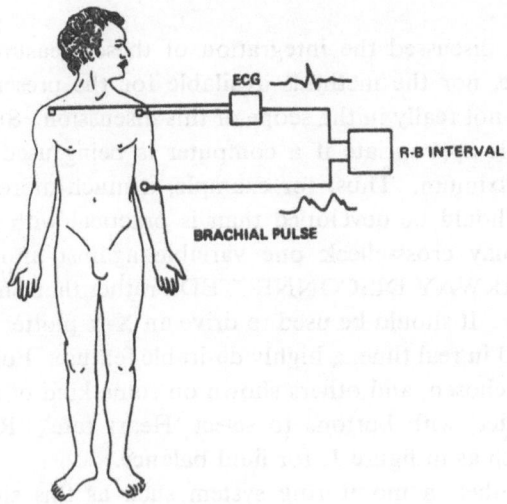

Fig. 8. Measurement of the R-B interval.

became shorter and shorter until she arrested – for a reason still unexplained. Though the anaesthetist had not detected anything abnormal, the R-B interval chart is clearly showing changes. She was successfully resuscitated with no sequelae.

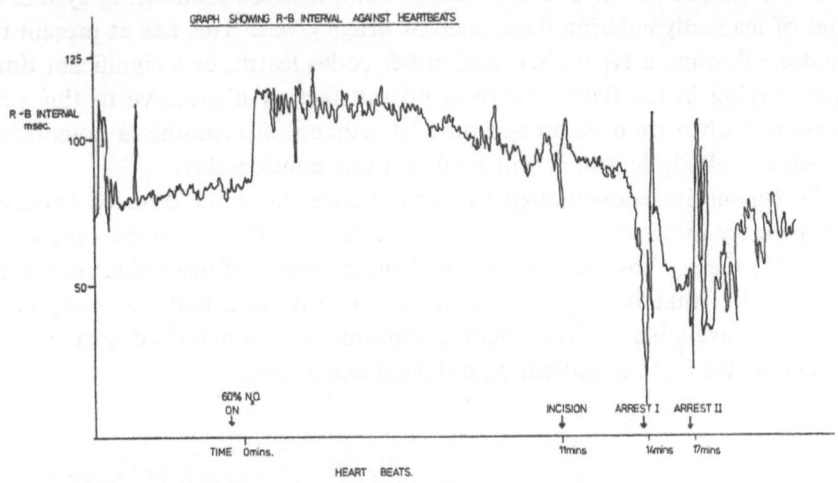

Fig. 9. R-B interval display during two cardiac arrests.

DISCUSSION

We have not yet discussed the integration of these measurements into a worthwhile whole, nor the methods available for the presentation of the results, for this is not really in the scope of this discussion. Suffice it to say, however, that it is appropriate if a computer is being used, to utilize its potential to a maximum. Thus, for example, a much more sophisticated warning system should be developed than is practical with purely analog methods. One may cross-check one variable against another, and for example warn 'AIRWAY DISCONNECTED', rather than show a red light or sound a buzzer. It should be used to drive an X-Y plotter generating an anaesthesia record in real time, a highly desirable feature. For this, selected variables may be chosen, and others shown on some kind of a display such as a scan converter, with buttons to select 'Heart rate', 'Respiration' or other charts – such as in figure 1, for fluid balance.

When put together, a monitoring system such as this significantly increases one's awareness of the clinical state of the patient. We have used one along these lines, and found that besides having untoward changes rapidly brought to our attention, what occurs is much better documented. It is frequently said that the vast majority of patients undergoing general anaesthesia develop cardiac arrhythmias. The heart rate display or the ECG waveform classification programs available will allow us to be much more precise about these clinical impressions. Also, the natural history of these arrhythmias and the need for and effect of therapy can be better documented.

The principal problem with a totally computerized monitoring system is that of manually entering data, such as drugs given. This has at present to be done through a typewriter, and either codes learnt, or a significant time spent typing in the data. There is no satisfactory alternative to this yet. However, when we have an accepted 'shorthand' of anaesthesia notetaking which everybody learns, it will facilitate this considerably.

To summarise, measurements in anaesthesia should be directed towards the primary indicators of the patient's status and those variables most influencing them. Absolute reliability of the system is of the highest concern. This implies that breakdowns must be very rare and that the equipment is always available. Given these conditions, a computerised system can be a valuable asset to patient care during anaesthesia.

ACKNOWLEDGEMENTS

I should like to acknowledge the invaluable help given by the Patient Monitoring Project team at Stanford University, California, in carrying out work contributing to this paper, and to Dr. C. Whitcher for data on the R - B interval. Work was funded by U.S. Health Services Grant No. HS 00146-03.

REFERENCES

1. Special committee investigating deaths under anaesthesia. Report of 745 classified cases, 1960—1968. *Med. J. Aust.* 1: 12, 573—592 (1970).
2. Bickford, R. G. Automatic EEG Control of General Anesthesia, E.E.G. Clin. Neuro. 2: 93-96 (1950).
3. Lowe, H. J, Dose regulated Penthrane Anesthesia Table 19, p. 91. Abbott Laboratories (1972).

COMPUTERS IN INTENSIVE THERAPY

JULIAN M. LEIGH

In intensive therapy, many systems of the body are of continuous and simultaneous interest so that the patient can be regarded as a data generator. The doctor and nurse can be regarded as the assimilators of this data, who process it, make decisions and feed an action or actions back into the patient's system, to determine the response. A repetition of this cycle of events may be required at frequent intervals. The large quantity of data generated during intensive therapy may be presented in an indigestible form and even with errors to the clinical team.

The utilisation of electronic methods of monitoring has done much to improve this situation, with the display of analogue waveforms and often of numerical displays of items such as blood pressures and pulse rate. However, the intensive therapy nurse still has to spend time keeping graphs, charting results of various blood parameters, and performing arithmetical operations on fluid balance information. The use of a digital computer and visual display system simplifies the data acquisition, improves the quality and accuracy of the data displayed and enables secondary mathematical manoeuvres to be carried out on the data (e.g. the calculation of urinary secretion rate, insensible perspiration rate and metabolic balance). Thus the quality of the information displayed to the team can be increased. In return for accuracy and standard chart production the nurse can concentrate more upon the patient.

Although there are computers around the world which control lung ventilators according to values of end-tidal carbon dioxide, tidal and minute volume, or control transfusion of fluids according to values of central venous pressure and arterial blood pressure, the philosophy that I adopt is that the computer should be used to perform tasks *very much better than humans can*, or preferably produce data in real time at the bedside, *which would otherwise be impossible to obtain*.

Figure 1 shows a diagrammatic representation of conventional management of a patient in intensive therapy. *Direct data* is obtained from the

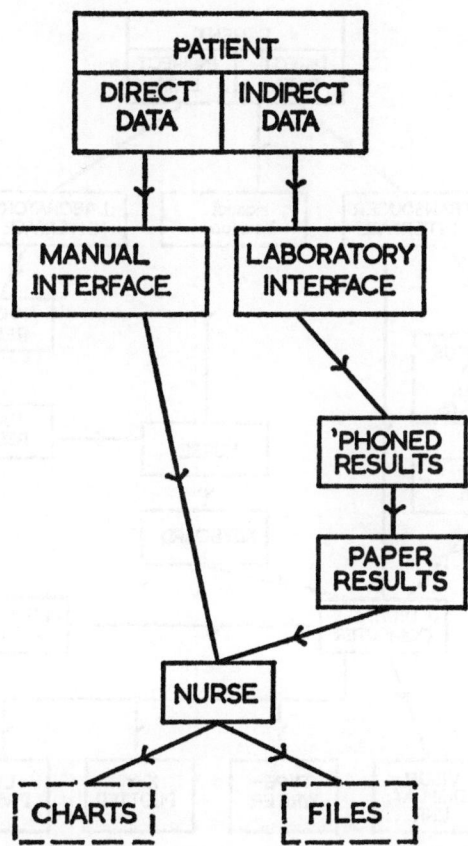

Fig. 1. Model of conventional patient management. The broken lines indicate the bedside facilities.

patient manually by the nurse and includes parameters such as temperature, blood pressure, pulse and respiration rates. *Indirect data* is obtained by sending samples from the patient to a laboratory where various estimations of parameters such as blood gases and electrolyte concentrations are made. All the data are finally collected together by the nurse, who may draw charts of physiological values and perform calculations of fluid balance, or she may place certain other data, such as biochemical results, into a file.

Figure 2 shows a model of patient management including a digital computer system and visual display unit (v.d.u.). Although this is superficially more complex, the bedside items are highlighted by the broken lines. It can be seen that a certain amount of direct data can be gathered automatically

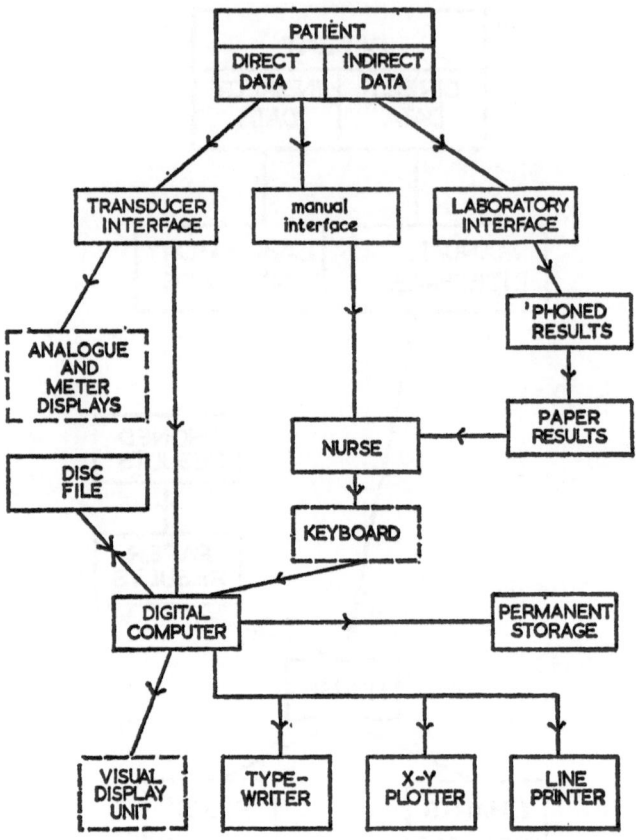

Fig. 2. Model of patient management including the computer system. The broken lines indicate the bedside facilities.

with electronic transducers, and the rest of the data can be input into the monitoring system by a nurse operating a hand-held keyboard. When the system is eventually completed the majority of the direct information will be transduced automatically. The nurse will be able to look after the needs of the patient and be able to call up any displays of relevant parameters on the v.d.u. by feeding in simple instructions from the keyboard.

COMPONENTS OF THE SYSTEM
The digital computer is an IBM 1800. The Ferranti visual display unit is under the control of a module which receives information from the computer and draws and refreshes the graphs on the screen. The keyboard

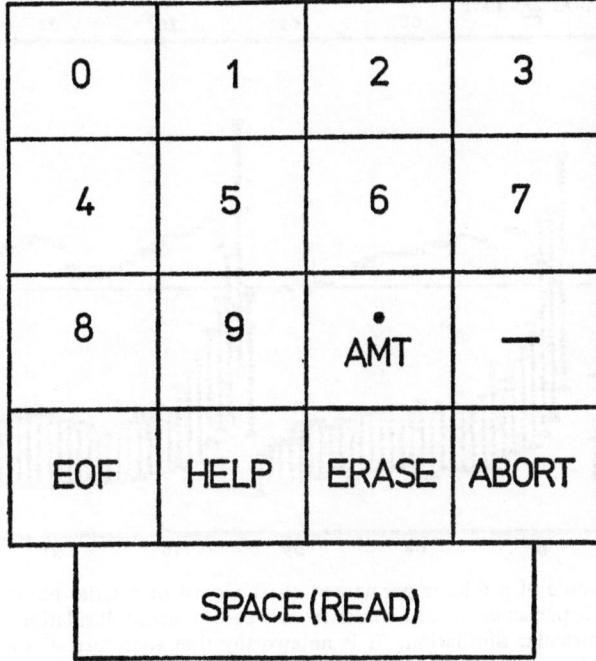

0	1	2	3
4	5	6	7
8	9	• AMT	—
EOF	HELP	ERASE	ABORT

SPACE (READ)

Fig. 3. Diagram of the seventeen key hand-held keybord for communicating with the system.

is shown diagrammatically in Figure 3 and has only seventeen keys. A small interface unit at the bedside enables the signals going directly to the computer to be switched off during manoeuvres such as physiotherapy, turning the patient, etc. In a side room of the Intensive Therapy Unit is an IBM typewriter on which 6-hourly charts are produced (Figure 4) for inclusion in the patient's notes, and on which half hourly brief summaries of current data are also typed in case of a system failure.

One limitation to application of this system is expense: at the moment we have only the bedside equipment to computerize three of the total complement of nine beds.

COMMUNICATING WITH THE SYSTEM

Communicating with the system involves two requirements, getting information in and getting processed information out.

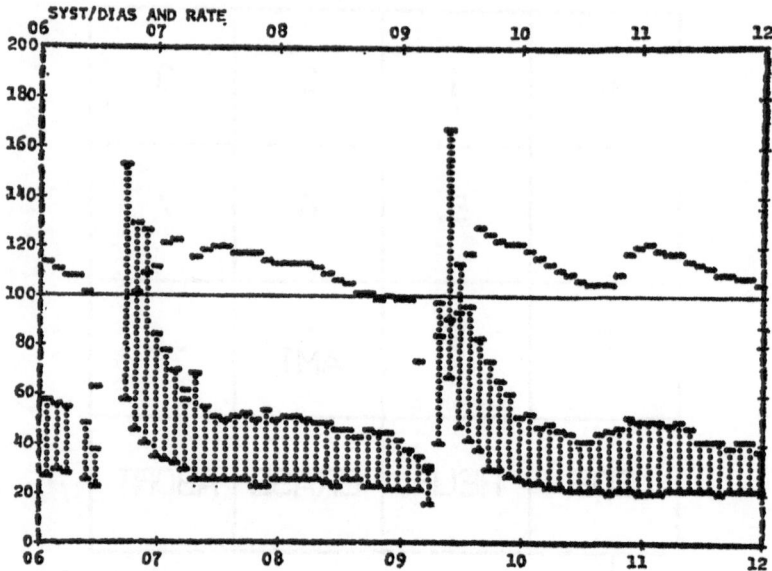

Fig. 4. An example of a 6-hour permanent chart record of arterial blood pressure and pulse rate. This particular record comes from a case of atrial fibrillation with two brief episodes of ventricular fibrillation. It is noteworthy that each 'arrest' was followed by relative arterial hypertension.

Information in

Where 'direct data' can be transduced automatically, it is preferable to do so. It is this interface technology which can be the limiting factor in the development of a fully automated system. In our system, blood pressures, pulse rates and temperature are transduced in a conventional manner, using both Statham and Hewlett Packard equipment. These parameters can also be entered manually if invasion of the patient is not felt justified. In this case the nurse fills in the numbers in a 'conversational mode' with the computer communicating via the keyboard and the v.d.u. Respiratory parameters, at the moment, are entered manually but electronic Wright's respirometers will be used in the near future for automatic monitoring.

At the present time fluid balance data is also entered manually, but in the future three types of transducers will also be used for automatic monitoring, i.e. infusion pump stepping motors with electrical output for transfusions and infusions, strain gauges for continuous weighing of drainage bags, and ultrasound for sensing drainage into cylindrical glass containers (working like SONAR) such as under-water seal chest drains.

With 'indirect data' the keyboard is the only method for getting the information into the system. However, in hospitals with autoanalysers under computer control, it may be possible in future for biochemical information to be communicated automatically to the system.

Fluid balance
Space does not permit by any means a full description of our system. However, the fluid balance section is worthy of some elaboration.

When basic values of fluid balance are entered, either automatically or manually, into the computer system calculations of fluid balance and metabolic data are accurately achieved. These also include the automatic continuous calculation of insensible perspiration losses based upon the patient's temperature, weight and height. Figure 5 shows the 'Fluid Logic Sequence' for getting the information into the system manually. As can be seen this is a branching system. Only the 'Fluids In', and 'Fluids Out', and '24 Hour Summaries' branches are fully programmed. The way in which this tree works is, if Code '60' is entered into the computer, the v.d.u. shows the five alternatives on the next row, one of which can be requested; and if 'Fluids In' or 'Fluids Out' are requested, a further 3 alternatives can be chosen.

Fluids in
Again, space does not permit a full description. However, to deal with

FLUID LOGIC SEQUENCE

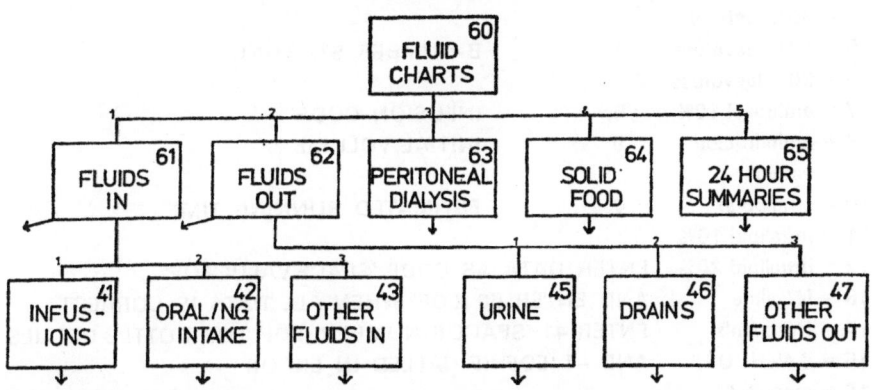

Fig. 5. Diagram showing the branching tree system used in the 'Fluid logic sequence' programmes.

'Infusions In': we had first to decide on how to identify infusion or transfusion bottles/bags for the computer. Normal charting usually consists of
a column for each drip, but as the fluid is going into the patient irrespective
of the route, it was decided to identify each separate bottle/bag by an infusion number or 'B-number', to be used in sequence, irrespective of which
drip was to be employed.

Figure 6 is the display obtained from Code 41 (see Figure 5), and is used
for changing infusions. On the left hand side can be seen a listing of infusion codes. If, for example, the infusion starting was normal saline, then
the keyboard entry would be 5 'Space' 13 'EOF'. By telling the computer
the volume and type of infusion, it knows the amounts of water, elec-
trolytes, calories, etc. that are given since these are programmed into the
system. These values are accumulated and the quantities given may be
obtained as a 24 hour metabolic summary.

The 'Estimated Running Time' enables the computer to continuously
update the fluid balance based upon the average infusion rate. This information can be over-ridden by updating the 'Volume Given So Far' on a

CHANGING INFUSION

CODE

1   TIME OF CHANGE   14.59

INFUSION CODES
 1 = blood   2   B-NUMBER FINISHED
 2 = plasma   3   FINAL VOLUME GIVEN
 3 = dextro-saline
 4 = 30% sorbitol
 5 = 10% laevulose   4   B-NUMBER STARTING
 6 = 20% laevulose
 7 = aminosol 10%   5   INFUSION CODE
 8 = amin.fruc.eth   6   INITIAL VOLUME
 9 = vamin
10 = aminoplex   7   ESTIMATED RUNNING TIME
11 = intralipid 10%
12 = intralipid 20%   ENTER DATA AS CODE 'SPACE'VALUE'EOF'
13 = N/saline   AND ENTER 66 'EOF' WHEN ALL DATA IS CORRECT
14 = Hartman's   ENTER 41 'SPACE'B-NUMBER 'EOF' FOR BOTTLE DETAILS
15 = 8.4%HCO3   AND −1 'EOF' IF CALLED IN ERROR
16 = mannitol

Fig. 6. Display used for 'Changing Infusion' – for full description see text.

further display of the relevant 'B number', or, in the future, will be over-ridden by directly transduced information from the infusion pumps.

Information out
Getting information out is a simpler problem, and is largely a matter of deciding what calculations should be made with the data, and how the processed information should be displayed. This depends on the limitations of the display system, and is also a matter of taste, since people differ as to whether they prefer numerical or graphical data, or a mixture of the two.

In general, we have chosen to produce numerical data only on '24 Hour Summaries' of fluid or metabolic balance. The bulk of the information is, however, displayed against time – either on a 6 hour or 18 hour time base – and, as will be seen, also includes *instantaneous* fluid balance information.

24 Hour summaries
Code 65 (see Figure 5) makes it possible to obtain this information for any previous 24 hour period and also the current incomplete day. For example, Figure 7 shows fluid balance data for 24 hours. It can be noted that different bottles/bags finished out of sequence and were therefore going into different drips. It is also noteworthy that the 'Fluid Out' column only contains actual positive entries so as not to distract attention; for instance, there is no line saying 'Nasogastric Aspirations' = zero.

FLUID BALANCE SUMMARY FOR 10.9

PATIENT NO.   O.   BED NO. 9

B-NUMBER	FLUID IN		FLUID OUT	
50	DEXTRO-SALINE	1000	URINE	2545
51	HARTMANS	450		
54	BLOOD	540		
53	BLOOD	540		
52	DEXTRO-SALINE	1000		
55	HARTMANS	1000		
56	DEXTRO-SALINE	275		
	TOTAL	4805	TOTAL	2545
FLUID BALANCE – 24 HOUR		2260	– OVERALL	2260

Fig. 7. 24 hour balance summary.

Graphical information

The clinician at the bedside manages his patient with respect to time and the information is therefore best displayed graphically.

A two digit code from the keyboard causes the display to list twelve alternatives, of which any three can be chosen (Figure 8). The display of no more than three of these at any one time is a limitation of the display system and is to a certain extent a disadvantage. However, relevant parameters can be easily selected according to the predominant interest of the patient. An illustrative record is shown in Figures 9a and b, which is from a case of bacteraemic shock. At the start of the record the patient was grey, cold and hypotensive with tachycardia, rapid respiration rate and oliguria. Treatment was given with infusions to maintain central venous pressure, with chlorpromazine and methyl-n-prednisolone for vasodilatation, frusemide to promote diuresis and lincomycin for the bacteraemia. At the end of the record the patient was pink and warm, with normal blood pressure, normal pulse rate, slower respiration rate and passing urine well.

BED NUMBER 4

SELECT THREE GRAPHS TO BE DISPLAYED
ENTER CODE 1 'SPACE' CODE 2 'SPACE' CODE 3 'EOF'

CODE	GRAPH
1	B.P. AND PULSE
2	VENOUS PRESSURES
3	TEMPERATURE
4	FLUID BALANCE
5	URINE RATE
6	URINE RATE M/K/H
7	BLOOD BALANCE
8	DRAIN RATE
9	DRAIN RATE M/K/H
10	MINUTE VOLUME
11	RESPIRATION RATE
12	TIDAL VOLUME

Fig. 8. Listing of twelve alternative graphical displays, of which any three can be viewed simultaneously.

Further development of these display graphs would include the indication of precise timing of interventions. For example, in Figure 9 it would be

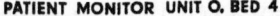

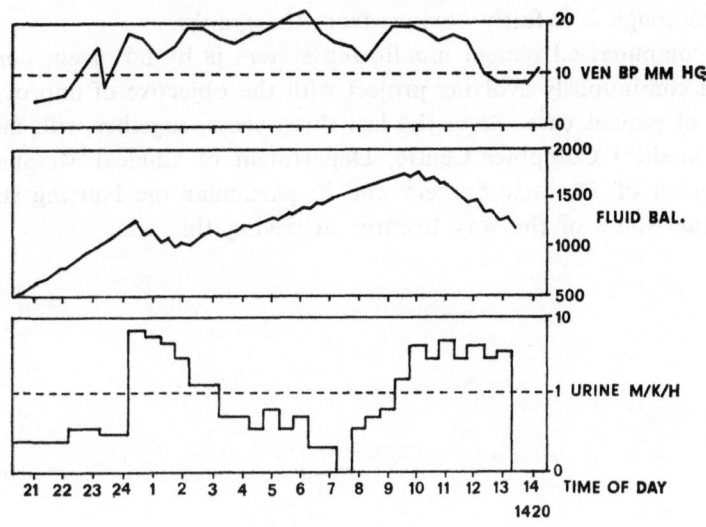

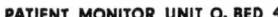

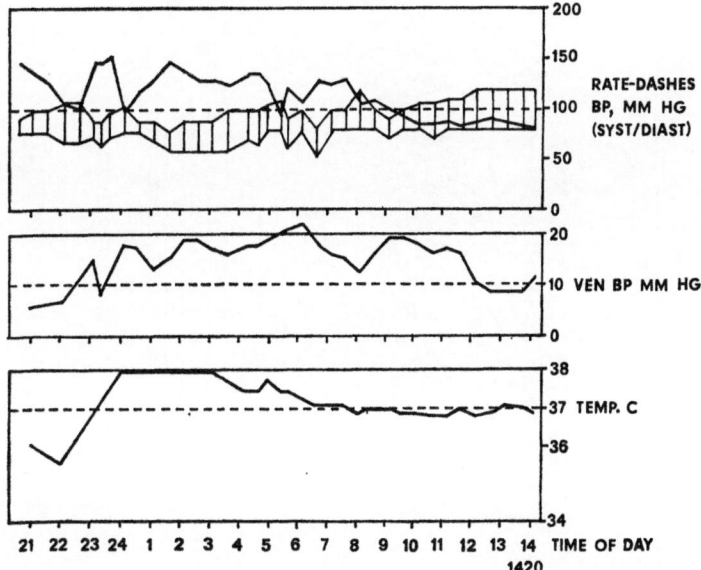

Fig. 9a and b. Eighteen hour record from a case of bacteraemic shock showing two displays, each of three graphs. The display of instantaneous fluid balance and urine secretion rate in ml/kg/hr (on a log scale) have proved particularly useful clinically (Fig. 9b).

advantageous to know precisely when the two doses of frusemide were given, although it is fairly obvious from the graphs.

Our computerised patient monitoring system is by no means complete, but is a continuously evolving project with the objective of improving the quality of patient care. Over the last three years, together with members of the Medical Computer Centre, Department of Clinical Measurement, Department of Thoracic Surgery and in particular the Nursing staff, we have gone some of the way towards achieving this aim.

INDEX OF SUBJECTS